Exercise Leadership in Cardiac Rehabilitation for High-Risk Groups

An Evidence-Based Approach

EDITED BY

Morag K. Thow, DIP PE, BSc, PhD, MCSP
Lecturer in Physiotherapy
Glasgow Caledonian University
Glasgow, UK

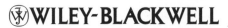

WILEY-BLACKWELL

A John Wiley & Sons, Ltd., Publication

This edition first published 2009
© 2009 John Wiley & Sons

Wiley-Blackwell is an imprint of John Wiley & Sons, formed by the merger of Wiley's global
Scientific, Technical and Medical business with Blackwell Publishing.

Registered office
John Wiley & Sons Ltd, The Atrium, Southern Gate, Chichester, West Sussex, PO19 8SQ,
United Kingdom

Editorial office
John Wiley & Sons Ltd, The Atrium, Southern Gate, Chichester, West Sussex, PO19 8SQ,
United Kingdom

For details of our global editorial offices, for customer services and for information about how to
apply for permission to reuse the copyright material in this book please see our website at
www.wiley.com/wiley-blackwell.

Library of Congress Cataloging-in-Publication Data

Cardiac rehabilitation exercises for high-risk groups: an evidence-based approach / edited by
Morag K. Thow.
   p. ; cm.
Includes bibliographical references and index.
ISBN 978-0-470-51512-9 (pbk.)   1. Heart–Diseases–Exercise therapy.   2. Heart–Diseases–Patients–
Rehabilitation.   3. Evidence-based medicine.   I. Thow, Morag K.
   [DNLM: 1. Heart Diseases–rehabilitation.   2. Evidence-Based Medicine.   3. Exercise
Therapy–methods.   4. Risk Factors.   WG 166 C26473 2009]
   RC684.E9.C373 2009
   616.1'203–dc22

                                                                                    2008049833

A catalogue record for this book is available from the British Library.

Set in 10/12pt Palatino by Aptara® Inc., New Delhi, India
Printed and bound in Singapore by Fabulous Printers Pte Ltd

1   2009

Contents

Contributors

Samantha Breen, MPhil, MCSP
Clinical Lead Physiotherapist, Surgical Office, Manchester Royal Infirmary, Manchester.

Samantha Breen is a clinical lead physiotherapist in cardiac rehabilitation and is the Chair of the Association of Chartered Physiotherapist in Cardiac Rehabilitation (ACPICR). She is involved in ACPICR development of standards, competencies, course development and delivery. She completed her MPhil in 2007, having researched cardiac rehabilitation provision in England. She is also a tutor and assessor on the BACR phase IV exercise instructor training programme and a member of the BACR subcommittee education steering group committee.

Mhairi Campbell, BSc, MCSP
Cardiac Rehabilitation Coordinator, Health at Heart Centre, Royal Alexandra Hospital, NHS Paisley, Paisley.

Mhairi Campbell has been involved in cardiac rehabilitation since 1997. Since 1999, Campbell has led the exercise aspect of the Scottish Demonstration Project 'Have a Heart Paisley', part of which has evaluated the menu-based approach to cardiac rehabilitation which is now accepted as the holistic approach to cardiac care.

Aynsley Cowie, BSc, MCSP
Senior 1 Physiotherapist, Ayr Hospital, Ayr.

Aynsley Cowie has been involved in developing and delivering cardiac rehabilitation in Ayrshire for a number of years. She is completing her PhD at Glasgow Caledonian University, undertaking an RCT on chronic heart failure and exercise. Aynsley has presented at many national and international forums on chronic heart failure.

Sue Dennell, Grad Dip Phys, MCSP
Transplant Physiotherapy Specialist, Cardiothoracic Transplant Unit, Wythenshawe Hospital, Wythenshawe, Manchester.

Sue Dennell has worked and taught in the field of cardiothoracic respiratory physiotherapy and cardiac rehabilitation for 28 years and has been involved with the transplant programme at Wythenshawe Hospital since its inception in 1987.

Hilary Dingwall, BSc, MCSP
Superintendent Physiotherapist, Cardiac Rehabilitation, Victoria Infirmary University NHS Glasgow, Glasgow.

Hilary Dingwall has worked in Cardiac Rehabilitation at the Victoria Infirmary for 12 years. She is actively involved in phases I–IV. Hilary was involved in the setting up of a Glasgow-wide cardiac rehabilitation ethnic minority service and has undertaken research into the frail elderly population, exercise and cardiac rehabilitation.

Patrick Doherty, PhD

Professor of Rehabilitation, Faculty of Health and Life Sciences, York St John University, York.

Professor Patrick Doherty is President of the BACR, National Clinical Lead for Cardiac Rehabilitation and continues to work clinically in York. Patrick has a special research interest in exercise in high-risk low capacity patients and has a number of PhD students researching the impact of seated exercise and resistance exercise in heart failure.

Alison Kirk, PhD

Lecturer in Sports Biomedicine, Institute of Sports and Exercise, University of Dundee, Dundee.

Dr Alison Kirk has a research expertise in physical activity promotion in people with type 2 diabetes in addition to development of theory-based physical activity behaviour change interventions, methods of physical activity measurement and physical activity in prevention and management of chronic disease. Alison has published and presented various research papers in these areas.

Lesley O'Brien, MSc, MCSP

Senior 1 Physiotherapist, Wishaw General Hospital, Motherwell.

Lesley O'Brien has been a senior physiotherapist in cardiac rehabilitation for 6 years. She has helped introduce a risk-stratified comprehensive cardiac rehabilitation programme offered to patients of variable risk and heart conditions. In conjunction with Lanarkshire CHD Managed Clinical Network, she has been involved in numerous projects including the implementation of a pan-Lanarkshire post-MI pathway.

Ann Taylor, PhD, MCSP

Head, Department of Physiotherapy, Faculty of Education and Health Sciences, University of Limerick, Ireland.

Dr Ann Taylor has an interest in the evidence base of cardiac rehabilitation, and was involved with the National Institute of Clinical Excellence in developing clinical guidelines for the management of people with chronic heart failure.

Morag K. Thow, PhD, MCSP

Lecturer in Physiotherapy, Glasgow Caledonian University, Glasgow.

Dr Morag K. Thow has been involved in the development and research of cardiac rehabilitation for over 25 years. She helped to establish the first exercise-based cardiac rehabilitation programme in Glasgow and continues to be involved in clinical education and research of cardiac rehabilitation.

Preface

Our first text *Exercise Leadership in Cardiac Rehabilitation* (Thow, 2006) fo-cused primarily on the more common patient groups of post-MI and revas-cularisation. We intentionally did not dedicate much of the first text to the pathophysiology of coronary heart disease and its presentations. In each of the chapters in this book, there is more of an emphasis on pathophysiology than in our first book. In addition, there is more emphasis on medications and other aspects that may be relevant to each group where applicable. This is because the patients that are the focus of this book are more com-plex and challenging. We have also included a chapter that embraces many of the copathologies that cardiac rehabilitation (CR) patients present with including the following:
- Peripheral arterial disease
- Arthritis
- Old age including hypertension

Many of the chapters in our first book *Exercise Leadership in Cardiac Rehabilitation* (Thow, 2006) are complementary to this text specifically the following:
- Chapter 3: Exercise physiology and monitoring
- Chapter 5: Class design and use of music
- Chapter 6: Leadership, exercise class management and safety
- Chapter 7: Teaching skills
- Chapter 8: Maintaining physical activity

Many of these chapters are relevant to the organisation and delivery of exercise to the conventional groups and these more complex groups in this text. We hope you find this text useful in developing and delivering your CR programmes.

Acknowledgements

I would like to acknowledge all the contributing authors who have been generous with their time, knowledge and experience. Also, I thank Dr Simon Williams, transplant and heart failure cardiologist, and Mr Nizar Yonan, cardiac transplant surgeon, for their contribution to Chapter 6. In addition, I thank Mrs Ann Ross and Mrs Bernie Downey for their contribution to Chapter 1. I also thank Dr Rowena Murray for her practical support and her encouragement to finish this book.

1   The Evolution of Cardiac Rehabilitation and Future Directions

Morag K. Thow

Chapter outline

There has been a dramatic development in medical and rehabilitative care for cardiac patient and family over the last 10–15 years in the UK. This chapter reviews the evolution of contemporary cardiac rehabilitation (CR) and the content of CR in the UK. The chapter also poses some questions and directions that CR may develop into the twenty-first century. This provides the context for the involvement of higher risk patients that this book addresses.

The evolution of cardiac rehabilitation

In the 1950s, CR consisted of extended periods of immobilisation, partic-ularly post-myocardial infarction (MI), for up to 6 weeks. The theory at that time was that reduced workload on the myocardium would allow myocardial healing. Furthermore, patients were informed that return to work and normal activity would be unlikely.

The pioneering work of Levine and Lown (1952) was innovative and radical for that time. In 1952 they introduced 'armchair management', where cardiac patients could recover by sitting for a period of 7 days, rather than the traditional bed rest that lasted up to 6 weeks. This early study of a more active approach to recovery after a cardiac event included 81 (16% women) 'post-coronary thrombosis' patients aged between 42 and 80 years. Levine and Lown were primarily interested in minimising the problems of bed rest and long periods of inactivity. It became clear that when the patients in this study were mobilised out of bed, stood up and took a few steps, their outcomes improved, or they at least had no more complications than before. Furthermore, the researchers claimed there were psychological benefits from early mobilisation, although they did not describe how these were measured.

Other clinicians in cardiac care at that time were becoming aware that extended immobility and bed rest were causing many psychologically and physiologically harmful effects. Newman *et al.* (1952) also encouraged an early 'active' approach to rehabilitation and had patients sitting, walking and stair climbing by their sixth week post-MI.

A further significant step was taken by Hellerstein and Ford in 1957. They advocated that not only was the traditional 'passive' bed rest approach detrimental to the rehabilitation of cardiac patients, but graded exercise should be included in the hospital phase along with early mobilisation. Although their early study was limited in that the exercise design was poorly described, their overall management post-event could be identified as one of the first comprehensive views of CR, as it included diet and stress management and other aspects of a holistic approach to a healthy life in their programme.

Once the misconception that inactivity was a requirement for recovery from a coronary event was dispelled in the 1950s, many researchers and clinicians started evaluating the effects of exercise for coronary heart disease (CHD) patients. This explosion of research was primarily driven by the growing evidence that not only was exercise post-event safe, there was compelling evidence that habitual exercise provided not only a measure of primary prevention (Morris *et al.*, 1953, 1966) but also secondary prevention benefits. The case for the possible benefits to CHD patients included in the work described by Hellerstein *et al.* (1967) who evaluated the physiological outcomes of 67 post-MI patients enrolled in a structured cycling exercise programme. The programme involved exercising three times per week for 4 months, training at a heart rate intensity of 150 beats/min. The researchers found a significant increase in work capacity and a significant reduction in the rate–pressure product. These findings from Hellerstein and colleagues' work, along with the work of others in the 1960s, were to change significantly the established cautious attitude to CHD patients and exercise.

In the early 1970s there was a dramatic change in attitude towards individuals who had CHD, and post-MI patients in particular. World leaders in exercise-based CR at this time included Kavanagh and Shephard (1973), who found that habitual structured exercise was not only safe after a coronary event but also afforded many physiological and psychological benefits. Thus, there was, in a 20-year period, a move away from the passive, and what we would now consider 'dangerous', bed rest for cardiac patients to an acceptance of early mobilisation and structured exercise as part of CR.

Cardiac rehabilitation in the UK in the early days

In 1970 Groden and colleagues carried out a survey of the then membership of the British Cardiac Society (BCS). One hundred sixty-four doctors replied. Findings revealed that 15% of them gave some advice about return to work and/or an advisory leaflet and 6% provided some form of exercise-based CR. Although there was very little comprehensive CR provision, one significant finding by Groden and colleagues (1970) was that 51% of the doctors who responded favoured development of CR in their units. Five years later, however, the Royal College of Physicians and the British Cardiac Society (RCP/BCS) (1975) reported that little had changed in the provision of CR. This report was not based on any new evidence, as they referred only to Groden *et al.* (1970). Like the 1970 survey the RCS report strongly supported the development of CR.

It took 12 years for any real developments in the UK. This occurred in 1987 with the London Symposium on 'Exercise-Heart-Health', hosted by the Coronary Prevention Group (CPG). This was followed by the establishment by the CPG of a committee led by Dr Hugh Bethell to address secondary prevention and rehabilitation. The first national conference, 'Recovering from a Heart Attack or Heart Surgery', was held in 1988 and was a great success, bringing together the supporters and advocates of CR.

The BCS report by Horgan *et al.* (1992) took a further significant step by making clear and important recommendations:
• Every major district hospital that treats patients with heart disease should provide a cardiac rehabilitation service.
• The programme should be multidisciplinary and usually exercise based.
                                              (Horgan *et al.*, 1992, p. 417).
This significant and extensive report identified that exercise of a suitably dynamic nature over a prolonged period up to 1 year could improve physiological outcomes, including central and peripheral cardiovascular adaptations. Furthermore, psychological outcomes could be improved, including elevation of mood and overcoming mild depression and anxiety (Horgan *et al.*, 1992). In addition, the report encouraged active involvement of the patient's family, especially in the educational aspect of CR, in order to support the adoption of other health-related behaviours. A more disappointing aspect of Horgan and colleagues' (1992) report was the continued lack of CR provision. They established that less than 50% of hospitals in the UK with cardiac units provided a CR programme. More disconcerting was the continued divergence of opinion among cardiologists and physicians about the potential for exercise-based CR to impact on physiological and psychological benefits. Horgan *et al.* (1992) emphasised this negative approach by some cardiologists to CR:

> The level of direct involvement by cardiologists in rehabilitation in the British Isles is very low, with less than one third of established CR courses retaining the support of the local cardiologist. It is perhaps surprising that although most cardiologists make extensive use of exercise testing after myocardial infarction, so few use this to aid exercise training. This may reflect the current emphasis in training on 'high-tech' procedures rather than a more holistic approach to patient care (Horgan *et al.*, 1992, p. 417).

There was reluctance by some cardiologists in the UK to accept the evidence that CR had potential physiological and psychosocial benefits for cardiac patients and families, but the tide was slowly turning. In concordance with the BCS (Horgan *et al.*, 1992) recommendations on CR provision, another eminent body, the Joint Cardiology Committee of the Royal College of Physicians endorsed CR in 1992:

> Cardiac rehabilitation should be available to all patients in the United Kingdom (Joint Cardiology Committee of the Royal College of Physicians, 1992, p. 106).

The British Association for Cardiac Rehabilitation (1992)

There was now considerable support for CR being generated in the UK. A historic development in CR occurred in September 1992, with a meeting of members of the CPG to establish a lead body for CR in the UK. This group produced the first constitution of the British Association for Cardiac Rehabilitation (BACR). The BACR was established in 1995 by some of the champions for CR, who recognised the need to provide a vehicle for galvanising those who had enthusiasm and belief in CR. It was intended to provide the first coordinated approach to CR in the UK, with the following aims:

• To promote a greater awareness and understanding of cardiac rehabilitation throughout the health care system.
• To facilitate communication and support among multidisciplinary professionals concerned with the rehabilitation of cardiac patients.
• To set national standards for cardiac rehabilitation and monitor the evaluation of these standards.
• To develop training programmes encompassing a multidisciplinary philosophy.
• To promote and facilitate research.
• To liaise with other national and international organisations working in this field.

(BACR, 1995, p. xiii).

The establishment of the BACR was a key development for cardiac care and rehabilitation in the UK. Until the BACR was established, CR practitioners were relatively isolated and had few forums for sharing or networking. The BACR filled a much-needed gap. In addition, since the inaugural meeting it has hosted an annual national conference, which gives members the opportunity to expand their network and hear about current research and best practice initiatives. The conference is a 2-day event that addresses current issues and incorporates eminent and acknowledged experts in the field of CR, such as Dr Stephen Blair, Dr Barry Franklin and Dr Erika Frolicher.

Publication of the 1995 BACR guidelines

The publication of the first BACR (1995) CR guidelines was a significant milestone for CR professionals. Until this important publication, CR professionals depended on evidence and guidelines from associations in other countries, primarily the US. The BACR guidelines were devised by experts working within CR at that time and provided a template for the UK to establish and deliver CR for a UK audience.

The 1995 BACR guidelines were produced by the early champions of CR, including Andrew Coates, Hanna McGee, Helen Stokes and David Thompson. The 13 expert contributors to the guidelines represented the multi-professional nature of CR. These guidelines provided purchasers and providers of CR with a working template to establish a comprehensive programme. The objective of the guidelines was to establish a benchmark for CR, which, for the first time in the UK, was based on the best available evidence at that time. The guidelines provided eight sections:

1. Historical background
2. Cardiac rehabilitation: programmes, content, management and administration
3. Medical aspects of CR
4. Exercise testing and prescription
5. Enhancing exercise motivation and adherence in CR
6. Psychosocial aspects of CR
7. Dietary aspects of CR
8. Funding issues in CR

The 1995 guidelines were a significant contribution to the expansion of effective and safe CR in the UK and continued to be highly relevant for practitioners into the early twenty-first century. Furthermore, as the UK 1995 guidelines were being launched, the World Council for Cardiac Rehabilitation was established, including Australia, Canada, South Africa and the US. Thus, the UK now had a forum, along with other associations, to promote and share research and good practice in order to enhance the provision of CR for all patients and families.

The authors of the 1995 guidelines acknowledged that they had only provided an overview of the available evidence. They had not carried out a full, 'in-depth' assessment of all aspects of CR.

National Service Framework for Coronary Heart Disease (2000)

In 2000 the National Service Framework (NSF) for CHD was published (DH, 2000). This was a further significant publication that acknowledged the place of CR in the management of heart disease. This ambitious document was the 'blueprint' for tackling CHD. It was developed by 38 experts and patient representatives in the field, chaired by Professor Sir George Alberti, President of the Royal College of Physicians, London. It aimed at

prevention, treatment and care for CHD patients in England. The document contained seven chapters (relating to 12 standards):
1. Reducing heart disease in the population (standards one and two)
2. Preventing CHD in high-risk patients (standards three and four)
3. Heart attack and other acute coronary syndromes (standards five, six and seven)
4. Stable angina (standard eight)
5. Revascularisation (standards nine and ten)
6. Heart failure (standard eleven)
7. Cardiac rehabilitation (Standard twelve)

(DH, 2000, p. 1).

The CR standards clearly set out the aim, rationale, effective interventions, service models, immediate priories, milestones and goals, holding the National Health Service (NHS) to account for their delivery:

> NHS Trusts should put in place agreed protocols/systems of care so that, prior to leaving hospital, people admitted to hospital suffering from coronary heart disease have been invited to participate in a multidisciplinary programme of secondary prevention and cardiac rehabilitation. The aim of the programme will be to reduce their risk of subsequent cardiac problems and to promote their return to full and normal life (DH, 2000, Ch. 7.0, p. 2).

As in the 1995 BACR guidelines, the NSF used the four phases of CR to describe the journey that cardiac patients should take through rehabilitation. Each phase gave clear guidelines on the intervention and care for that phase. Phase III included structured exercise sessions delivered to meet the assessment needs of individual patients. The NSF recommended the following:

> Exercise sessions may be structured in a variety of ways to meet the needs of individual patients. Typically they will be provided to groups, last at least 6 weeks, but normally 12 weeks or more and comprise at least 3 sessions per week with a minimum of 2 supervised exercise sessions (individual programmes often in a group environment) and 1 session of education and information for patients, partners, carers and families (DH, 2000, Ch. 7.0, p. 5).

The NSF CR standard recommended exercise as part of phase III and into phase IV, but the content and delivery of the exercise sessions were not fully described. The standard acknowledged that considerable lifestyle change is required by cardiac patients and families in order to reduce coronary risk. In addition to exercise, education, lifestyle, vocational and psychological support is part of comprehensive CR. Thus, this document embedded CR within comprehensive care for cardiac patients and families.

Scottish Intercollegiate Guideline Network Guideline (2002)
Early in 2000 the Scottish Intercollegiate Guideline Network (SIGN) was commissioned to produce a guideline on CR. SIGN is a collaborative

network of clinicians, health professionals and patient organisations. It is funded by the Clinical Resource and Audit Group (CRAG) of the Scottish Executive Health Department. Guideline for SIGN is developed by multidisciplinary teams invited to be part of the development group. The chairman of the group was Dr Chris Isles, a consultant physician, who invited 18 expert members to form the development group. Like the BACR, they represented the multi-professional nature of CR.

All SIGN expert groups use a standard methodology to provide systematic review of the available evidence. For the SIGN 2002 CR guideline, all evidence up to 2000 was systematically synthesised by members of the group. The evidence for a SIGN guideline is based only on publications that adhere to recognised scientific principles of methodology, including sample size, clear hypothesis and outcomes and accurate reporting of the results. The SIGN 2002 CR guideline drew on peer-reviewed papers, systematic reviews and meta-analysis, including Jolliffe *et al.* (2000), Goble and Worcester (1999) and Oldridge *et al.* (1988). Once the SIGN group produces the draft guideline, further rigorous consultation and peer-reviewing process follows. For the CR guideline a national open meeting was held in March 2001, and comments were gathered from key specialists attending the meeting. In addition, the SIGN 57 CR guideline was made available on the SIGN website for further comment. Lastly, 20 independent expert referees were canvassed for comment on the accuracy and completeness of the interpretation of the available evidence supporting the recommendations in the guideline.

The main difference in the SIGN 2002 CR guideline from the first BACR 1995 guideline was that evidence and recommendations were assigned grades and levels of evidence. These were based on the quality and amount of available evidence. The recommendations for each section and subsection identified were given a grade, from A to D, with supplementary good practice points. The SIGN 57 2002 CR guideline contained 12 A recommendations, 9 B, 2 C, 8 D and 9 good practice points. The SIGN CR 57 guideline was published in January 2002. It was supported and endorsed by the BACR as a national UK guideline. Thus, it superseded the 1995 BACR guideline.

Although there had been definitions of CR in the past, in other publications the SIGN group identified key elements in CR. The authors also acknowledged the involvement of family, partners and carers in the rehabilitation process. The following definition was provided:

> Cardiac rehabilitation is the process by which patients with cardiac disease, in partnership with a multidisciplinary team of health professionals, are encouraged and supported to achieve and maintain optimal physical and psychosocial health (SIGN, 2002, p. 1).

This definition is still relevant today and is applicable in the present CR context. When this definition was proposed, the majority of patients entering CR programmes, with a few exceptions, were post-acute myocardial infarction (AMI) and had experienced revascularisation procedures, including coronary artery bypass grafting (CABG).

The SIGN guideline comprised eight sections:

1. Introduction

Remit and definitions, four phases of CR, need for a guideline, current provision, uptake and review and updating

2. Psychological and educational interventions

Psychological predictors of risk, measurement of psychosocial well-being, effectiveness of psychosocial and educational interventions, principles of behaviour change, educational and psychosocial interventions and aspects of behavioural change

3. Exercise training

Benefits of exercise training, safety issues, assessment before exercise training, staffing, location, exercise content, monitoring of exercise training, resistance training and long-term exercise training

4. Interventions in specific patient groups

Post-MI, post-coronary bypass and angioplasty, stable angina, chronic heart failure, older patients, women, other groups

5. Long-term follow-up

Transition to primary care, follow-up in primary care, shared care, self-help groups and long-term exercise programmes

6. Information for patients and professionals

Notes for discussion with patients, sources of further information

7. Implementation and audit

Statement of intent, implementation, resource implications of implementing the guidelines, audit

8. Development of the guideline

The guideline development group, systematic literature review, consultation and peer review.

Although SIGN in 2002 acknowledged that more complex and higher risk groups had the potential to benefit from CR programmes, there was less evidence for these groups. However, since then, with publication of our first text *Exercise Leadership in Cardiac Rehabilitation* (Thow, 2006), a significant body of evidence has developed, acknowledging that CR is safe and effective for these other groups. Thus, in 2008 not only is there an increase in the number of 'conventional' patients in CR, but there is also a need to integrate higher risk groups into CR programmes.

One point of note in the SIGN guideline was that the section on Exercise Training and Long-Term Exercise Programme comprised the largest part of the publication. This reinforced the important contribution exercise has to make in terms of the cardioprotective effects of habitual exercise in CR. Furthermore, this section, unlike the NSF 2000 publication, provided exercise professionals with guidelines on the assessment, monitoring and content of the exercise component of CR.

BACR Standards and Core Components for Cardiac Rehabilitation (2007)

This standards document was developed by 16 experts, primarily working or associated with CR in the UK. The group was co-chaired by Professor Patrick Doherty and Mrs Bernie Downey. The standards were devised to assure the BACR membership and the public that agreed best practice is available to all eligible patients. The 2007 standards replaced any previous standards, and the recommended six minimum standards in this document were to be audited from data that the National Audit of Cardiac Rehabilitation (NACR) would gather. The standards group advised that the standards be reviewed in 2010.

For these six standards, each must achieve core requirements:
- A coordinator who has overall responsibility for the CR service
- A CR core team of professionally qualified staff with appropriate skills and competencies to deliver the service
- A standard assessment of individual patient's needs
- Referral and access for targeted patient population
- Registration and submission of data to the NACR
- A CR budget appropriate to meet the full service cost

(BACR, 2007, p. 2).

This thorough standards document outlines the content and components for CR. This document interestingly does not describe CR in the traditional phases of CR. It will be interesting to see in the future, when the NACR audit database is measured, if CR across the UK reaches these 'minimum' standards and core components.

Service Framework for Cardiovascular Health and Wellbeing (2008)

The recent consultation document, Service Framework for Cardiovascular Health and Wellbeing (SFCHW, 2008), by the Department of Health, Social Services and Public Safety for Northern Ireland, is a far-reaching document, led by Dr David Stewart. It was developed by 25 members of a broad range of clinicians, service users and carers. In addition, like the NSF (2002) standard, these standards should be measurable.

Several of the standards in this document are condition specific, with CHD being one condition. The service framework embraces prevention, diagnosis, treatment, care, rehabilitation and palliative care of both individuals and communities who have greater risk of developing cardiovascular disease (CVD). Standard 24 includes CR:

All patients identified as requiring cardiac rehabilitation, in line with the British Association for Cardiac Rehabilitation guidelines, should be offered this service. Percentage of patients eligible for cardiac rehabilitation who receive the components of the service based on assessment of their need March 2009–60%, March 2010–70%, March 2011–85% (SFCHW, 2008, p. 17).

It will be interesting to see, in the future, how this extensive and ambitious project impacts on the cardiovascular health and well-being of the Northern Ireland population. Furthermore, of more interest will be the demand and need for comprehensive menu-based CR in Northern Ireland in the future.

Content of contemporary CR

The SIGN 2002 and NSF 2000 guidelines identified four phases of CR, progressing from the early hospital admission stage to long-term maintenance of lifestyle changes:
- Phase I – Inpatient period or after a 'step change' in cardiac condition
- Phase II – Early post-discharge
- Phase III – Supervised outpatient programme including structured exercise
- Phase IV – Long-term maintenance of exercise and other lifestyle changes

(SIGN, 2002, p. 2).

Phase I

Phase I is recognised as the first point of contact within the acute setting. It is considered to be either the inpatient stage or after a 'step change' in the patient's cardiac condition. A step change may include presentation of an MI, cardiac surgery, angioplasty/stent and acute coronary syndrome, first diagnosis of heart failure (McKenna and Forfar, 2002; SIGN, 2002). In this phase, patients may be anxious and/or depressed regarding the threat to their health. It is important that support and reassurance are given by the CR team, with misconceptions being addressed (SIGN, 2002).

Phase I CR has traditionally included assessment, education, risk stratification and exercise/mobilisation. Assessment involves identifying risk factors and risk stratification, with the educational aspect providing patients with appropriate individual information regarding CHD, risk factors and lifestyle (Proudfoot *et al.*, 2007; SIGN, 2002). The patients and families are prepared for transition to phase II, and links are made with the phase III team. This stage is a short phase of approximately 3–4 days, or until the patient is stabilised. Other early interventions include the 'Heart Manual', a 6-week comprehensive home-based programme that has been well evaluated and is especially useful in rural locations (Lewin *et al.*, 1992).

Phase II

This is the early post-discharge stage back to the community and home. It is a time when patients feel isolated and insecure, and when high levels of anxiety may be present in both patient and family. To minimise this psychological impact of return home, the CR team can maintain contact by phone or home visit. Furthermore, the primary care team may also be involved at this stage and can minimise the impact. This is the stage where early modification of risk factors will start and goals set in phase I CR should start

have endorsement from a phase II exercise professional and a character reference. This prestigious course is recognised by the Register of Exercise Professionals, Skills Active, BHF and the BCS and contributes significantly to the participants' continuing professional development (CPD).

The BACR phase IV has administrative support from two full-time members of staff. Over the last 11 years, 40 BACR tutors have been trained. The material delivered includes a standardised course manual, accompanying DVD and workbooks. The course is delivered UK-wide in ten regional centres. The content of the course includes 5 days, 35 hours contact, 100 hours of independent study and a visit to a phase III programme. The students have one day to review and prepare assessment material. The assessment is carried out over a half-day and includes a written multiple-choice question paper, a written case study and a viva. Every 3 years students are required to revalidate their qualification with a 1-hour paper and evidence of working with phase IV participants. Once the students qualify, they automatically become members of the BACR phase IV instructors' network.

In 2006 a survey was carried out on the provision of phase IV in the UK (Thow *et al.*, 2006). Of the BACR phase IV members, 498 from 800 (63%) members replied to a postal survey. The main findings of the survey were that 65% of programmes were held in a community setting, and referrals from phase III constituted over 75%. Weekly, there were over 600 classes in the UK, with approximately 12 000 participants exercising in phase IV. The more negative outcome of the study highlighted the disparity of funding across the UK: some areas had good support from NHS sources (28%) and leisure services (24%), while the rest were self-funding and less financially secure. There was overwhelming support for the BACR course providing a quality educational experience by 80% of the respondents. This course has been one of the most significant and valuable contributions to ongoing care in CR in the UK.

Association of Physiotherapists in Cardiac Rehabilitation
The ACPICR is acknowledged by the Chartered Society of Physiotherapy (CSP) as a clinical interest group for physiotherapists in CR. This group is affiliated to the BACR. The group was established in 1995 and was called initially the *Association of Physiotherapists Interested in Cardiac Rehabilitation*. This organisation has a dynamic committee and regional representatives contributing to the national body. In 2008 the membership of ACPICR was 169, with 139 physiotherapists and the rest of the membership being a variety of professionals and exercise professionals.

The ACPICR has been proactive in liaising with organisations and government bodies that are the key drivers for CR, including the NICE guideline groups and national audit groups. The APICR also contributes to the CSP annual conference, thus providing a high profile for CR professionals. In collaboration with the CSP, in 2006 the iCSP website was established for the APICR interest group. This site provides exchange and dissemination of research across the membership. The website for CR 2006 had over 1600 users, thus showing the extent of interest in CR.

To further the objectives of the ACPICR, the group produced a comprehensive guideline handbook for the delivery of phase III exercise-based CR, *The Standards for the Phase III Exercise Component of Cardiac Rehabilitation* (ACPICR, 1999, 2006). (This guideline is presently being updated.) This user-friendly guideline is evidence based and provides CR physiotherapists with up-to-date best practice guidelines for safe and effective design and delivery of CR. It was endorsed by the BACR in 2007 as part of the core competencies of CR.

In addition to the guidelines, the ACPICR produced competencies for physiotherapists involved in the care and management of CHD patients attending exercise-based phase III CR (ACPICR, 2005, 2008a) (to be updated in 2010). The authors of the competency document give the following rationale for the document:

> The overall aim is to provide clear guidelines about the expected role, standards of performance and the knowledge and skills required to achieve quality care for the exercise component of Phase III CR (ACPICR, 2008a, p. 2).

To support the delivery of the competencies, a peer review booklet was published by the ACPICR (2008b). The booklet supports peer observation of the actual delivery of the phase III exercise CR. It uses a 'traffic light' system to reflect if the standards are achieved, partly achieved or not achieved. The ACPIC interest group is one of the most dynamic and proactive within the CSP, in relation to the production of evidence-based guidelines and methods to help members maintain quality and standards.

The ACPICR is key deliverer of quality CPD courses in the UK for those delivering exercise-based CR. The courses are held over 1 or 2 days, and in 2007 the courses included the following:
• Exercise prescription, new insights and management of the complex patient
• Skills and techniques in delivering group exercise
• A practical course in assessing and monitoring functional capacity in cardiac patients
• Assessment, prescription and delivery of physical activity for the patient with heart failure, a nurse professional study day and an exercise professional study day.

Furthermore, the ACPICR informs the membership through the newsletter and website of validated MSc modules and courses across the UK. In 2008 over 20 academic institutions in the UK were delivering validated MSc and modular courses for CR professionals. These institutions offer a mixture of single modules or full MSc in CR.

Exercise Professionals' Group
The ACPIC, BACR and the British Association of Sports and Exercise Science (BASES) make up the Exercise Professionals' Group (EPG),

established in 2003. Other EPG members are graduate members of the BACR phase IV graduate network of over 800 graduates. This group has a yearly study day where updates in current research and developments in exercise delivery in CR are provided. All members of the phase IV graduate group receive a newsletter from the BACR. An exciting development was a pilot psychology course in 2006, with the first full course taking place in June 2008. The course is still in the developmental stage. In addition, this group is in the developmental stages of running an Introduction to Cardiac Rehabilitation for commissioners and new clinicians to the field.

Cardiac rehabilitation future directions

Since the early work of CR pioneers, over 50 years ago, we can see a massive change in attitudes to the management of cardiac patients. Furthermore, there has been a massive shift in the UK to the 'active' approach to rehabilitation. Early exercise and holistic management are now the norm, but how will CR develop in the near and distant future?

High-risk groups

Many patients in the 1950s and up to a few years ago were either excluded from CR, due to their apparent 'high risk' or by reluctant clinicians, who did not feel equipped to deal with higher risk groups. These 'high-risk' patients, with the increase in evidence and quality research, are more likely now to be included in comprehensive menu-based CR. In the future, will we see most, if not all, of the 'lower risk' patients, for example, uncomplicated MI CABG, moved quickly into community-based phases III and IV CR and increased CR for 'high-risk' groups in the hospital setting? This text addresses these questions.

Mentoring and self-help groups

With the projected increase in the numbers of patients accessing CR and the need for ongoing health behaviour change, there could be more expansion and use of lay health mentoring to empower people with CHD and CVD. There have been successful examples of this approach to empowerment, where support and advice are given by peers who have experienced CHD. The Braveheart Project in Falkirk, Scotland, for older people with ischaemic heart disease is one such example (Coull *et al.*, 2004). This randomised controlled trial, over 1 year, with 289 participants aged 60 years and over diagnosed with MI or angina, found significant improvements in the mentored group in exercise participation, improved diet, improved concordance with medication, physical functioning on the SF-36 score and reduced outpatient attendance for CHD. The authors of this innovative approach found that the approach is feasible, safe and inclusive, positively influenced lifestyle, in particular exercise and diet, complements CR and, finally, is a model that can achieve measurable health gains. A similar project with older people, designed to increase exercise participation, has seen a similar mentoring programme influence over 12 000 older people to increase exercise (Laventure *et al.*, 2008). It could be possible in the future to utilise this approach more in order to maintain exercise and healthy lifestyle.

Is it cardiovascular rehabilitation and/or prevention?

As discussed earlier, CR patients in the past were primarily from the lower risk post-MI and CABG groups. Now we are seeing more complex and higher risk groups. As CHD is only one manifestation of CVD, there is a clear overlap of patients presenting to CR with diabetes, peripheral vascular disease and transient ischaemic attacks. Many CR patients present with many of these conditions. As we will see in Chapters 2 and 6 of this text, type 2 diabetes and peripheral vascular disease are common among CR patients. Fitzgerald-Barron (2005) acknowledges the overlap in disease management and that CR patients share many common cardiovascular risks and need cardiovascular management. It is also of interest that BACR and 15 other affiliate groups are now part of the British Cardiovascular Society. The National Service Framework for Coronary Heart Disease in England comes to an end in 2009/2010 and there is currently no strategy to replace it. The Cardio & Vascular Coalition will see in England a campaigning for a new comprehensive Cardio & Vascular Health Strategy for 2010–2020. In the future, will we see CR become a broader remit to embrace all patients with CVD?

Furthermore, will prevention of CVD become a strategy as in Northern Ireland (SFCHW, 2008)? Will proactive involvement in prevention, promotion, protection and lifestyle become the remit of the CR team? Should rehabilitation move into prevention and become more proactive in order to prevent patients who are at high risk of CHD developing CHD?

Will cardiac rehabilitation phases be redundant?

The concept of phases of CR traditionally represents parts of the journey that cardiac patients take in their pathway of care. It could be argued that the phases represent only where the patient is. For example, phase I is in hospital, phase II is at home, phase III is back in structured exercise and, lastly, phase IV is lifetime maintenance at home. These phases in the SIGN (2002) definition are not intended to relate simply to location, but are intended to tailor interventions to the individual.

Although SIGN (2002) suggests that CR is menu based, perhaps compartmentalising CR into phases is not the best design. The design at present, especially phases I–III, lasts approximately 3–4 months. However, it could be agued that this amount of time is too short to impact on behaviour change and to accrue the health benefits of exercise. Other programmes have contact with patients for much longer periods, for example, up to 1 year (Kavanagh *et al.*, 2008). Should rehabilitation be structured in the UK to have a longer contact period, especially in the present phase III, where the support and behaviour change is at the most intense? Other 'packages' of CR could be devised, such as the following two examples:

1. A 6-month phase III programme: the first 2 months (two classes per week plus one home session), followed by 4 months (one class per month plus home session and continued support calls from the CR team). This represents 20 CR contact sessions spread over 6 months, compared to the current model of 12-week phase III class of two sessions, providing 24 contacts. Another advantage of this model is that the patient is gradually being given more responsibility and increased self-management. With behaviour change strategies running over a longer period of time, not only there may be improved adherence and improved self-efficacy, but the transition to phase IV may also be smoother.

2. Instead of having phases, subjects stay in the CR programme till they reach agreed milestones or goals, for example, are able to safely self-monitor, achieve agreed BMI/waist-to-hip ratios, achieve a 6 metabolic equivalents shuttle walk test result. It could be argued that CR, particularly phase III, is not flexible to the CR individual's goals. It would be interesting to shape a programme around goals and targets for the patient.

Key messages

- CR is now firmly embedded in cardiac care in the UK.
- The BCS, BACR and other affiliated groups have developed and led an enormous development in quality, evidence-based CR.
- There will be a substantial increased demand for CR if the targets set by national government are achieved.
- Not only will there be more demand for low- and moderate-risk CR patients, there will be more high-risk patients included in CR.
- CR is continually evolving and improving, due to research and evidence-based practice.
- There may be extended development and use of self-help and mentoring programmes to expand and support CR.
- In the future, CR may encompass all cardiovascular groups and move more into primary prevention.

Summary

In the 1950s pioneering work explored a more active approach to the rehabilitation of cardiac patients. These early developments in CR laid the foundations for others in the 1960s–1970s to devise more structured exercise-based programmes that began to turn the tide not only in attitudes but also in building the evidence base for CR. The establishment of the BACR as the lead body for CR was a significant development in the UK. This group was the first to galvanise, provide direction and a communication framework for CR professionals. Since then, CR is now firmly embedded in cardiac care, with over 370 CR programmes in the UK. CR is now supported by education and CPD from the BACR and affiliated groups and many universities across the UK, providing quality MSc and standalone modules in CR. Furthermore, there has been much quality research on the many facets of CR, which continues to shape and improve the care for CR recipients. A major shift in the twenty-first century is that the previously branded 'high-risk' patients, which this book explores, can safely be included in exercise-based CR. In addition, new forms of CR are emerging: Will we see in the future increased utilisation of mentoring and self-help by ex-patients and those with CVD to empower them to change and maintain health cardiovascular behaviour? CR is still evolving. The future of CR provision may see a move towards different 'packaging' of CR, possibly embracing CVD prevention.

References

Association of Chartered Physiotherapists in Cardiac Rehabilitation (ACPICR) (1999) *Standards for the Exercise Component of Phase III Cardiac Rehabilitation.* London: CSP.

Association of Chartered Physiotherapists in Cardiac Rehabilitation (ACPICR) (2005, 2008a) *Competencies for the Exercise Component of the Phase III Cardiac Rehabilitation.* London: CSP.

Association of Chartered Physiotherapists in Cardiac Rehabilitation (ACPICR) (2006) *Standards for the Exercise Component of Phase III Cardiac Rehabilitation.* London: CSP.

Association of Chartered Physiotherapists in Cardiac Rehabilitation (ACPICR) (2008b) *Peer Review for the Exercise Component of the Phase III Cardiac Rehabilitation.* London: CSP.

Bethell, H.J.N., Turner, S.C., Evans, J.A.R., *et al.* (2001) Cardiac rehabilitation in the United Kingdom: how complete is the provision? *Journal of Cardiopulmonary Rehabilitation*, 21, 111–15.

Borg, G.A.V. (1982) Psychophysical bases of perceived exertion. *Medicine and Science in Sports and Exercise*, 14, 377–81.

British Association for Cardiac Rehabilitation (BACR) (1995) *BACR Guidelines for Cardiac Rehabilitation.* Oxford: Blackwell Science.

British Association for Cardiac Rehabilitation (BACR) (1999) *Cardiac Rehabilitation: An Educational Resource.* Colourways Ltd.

British Association for Cardiac Rehabilitation (BACR) (2002) *Phase IV Exercise Training Module.* Leeds: Human Kinetics.

British Association for Cardiac Rehabilitation (BACR) (2007) *Standards and Core Components for Cardiac Rehabilitation.* Available from http://www.bcs.com (accessed 10 April 2007).

British Heart Foundation (BHF) (2006) *British Heart Foundation: Heart Disease Statistics Database.* London: British Heart Foundation. Available from http://www.heartstats.org (accessed 5 February 2007).

Coull, A.J., Taylor, V.H., Elton, R., *et al.* (2004) A randomised controlled trial of senior lay health mentoring in older people with ischaemic heart disease: The Braveheart Project. *Age and Ageing*, 33, 348–54.

Department of Health (2000) *The Coronary Heart Disease: National Service Frameworks for Coronary Heart Disease*. London: Department of Health.

Fitzgerald-Barron, M. (2005) Setting a pace in cardiac rehabilitation. *The British Journal of Cardiology*, 12(5), 329–30.

Goble, A.J., Worcester, M.U.C. (1999) *Best Practice Guidelines for Cardiac Rehabilitation and Secondary Prevention*. Melbourne: The Heart Research Centre.

Groden, B.M., Semple, T., Shaw, G.B. (1970) Cardiac rehabilitation in Britain. *British Heart Journal*, 33, 756–8.

Hellerstein, H.K., Ford, A.B. (1957) Rehabilitation of the cardiac patient. *Journal of the American Medical Association*, 164, 225–31.

Hellerstein, H.K., Hornstein, T.R., Goldbarg, A., *et al.* (1967) The influence of active conditioning upon subjects with coronary artery disease. *Physical Activity and Cardiovascular Health*, 96, 758–9.

Horgan, J., Bethell, H., Carson, P. (1992) Working party report on cardiac rehabilitation. *British Heart Journal*, 67, 462–8.

Joint Cardiology Committee of the Royal College of Physicians (1992) Provision of services for the diagnosis and treatment of heart disease. *British Heart Journal*, 67, 106–16.

Jolliffe, J.A., Rees, K., Taylor, R.S., *et al* (2000) Exercise-based rehabilitation for coronary heart disease. *Cochrane Database for Systematic Reviews* 1. CD001800. Available from http://www.cochrane.org (accessed 14 February 2007).

Kavanagh, T., Hamm, L.F., Beyene, J., *et al.* (2008) Usefulness of improvement in walking distance versus peak oxygen uptake in predicting prognosis after myocardial infarction and/or coronary artery bypass graft in men. *The American Journal of Cardiology*, 101(10), 1423–27.

Kavanagh, T., Shephard, R.J. (1973) Importance of physical activity in post-coronary rehabilitation. *American Journal of Physical Medicine*, 52, 3304–13.

Laventure, R.M.E., Dinan, S.M., Skelton, D.A. (2008) Someone like me: increasing participation in physical activity among seniors with senior peer health motivators. *Journal of Aging and Physical Activity*, 16, S76–7.

Levine, S.A., Lown, B. (1952) Armchair treatment of acute coronary thrombosis. *Journal of the American Medical Association*, 148, 1365–9.

Lewin, B., Robertson, I.H., Cay, E.L., *et al.* (1992) Effects of self-help post myocardial infarction rehabilitation on psychological adjustment and use of health services. *Lancet*, 339(1), 1036–40.

McKenna, C.J., Forfar, J.C. (2002) Was it a heart attack? *British Medical Journal*, 324, 377–8.

Morris, J.N., Healey, J.A., Raffle, P.A.B., *et al.* (1953) Coronary heart-disease and physical activity of work. *Lancet*, 2, 1150–57, 1111–20.

Morris, J.N., Kagan, A., Pattison, D.C., *et al.* (1966) Incidence and prediction of ischaemic heart-disease in London busmen. *Lancet*, 2, 553–9.

Newman, L.B., Andrews, M.F., Koblish, M.O., *et al.* (1952) Physical medicine and rehabilitation in acute myocardial infarction. *Archives of Internal Medicine*, 89, 552–61.

Oldridge, N.B., Guyatt, G.H., Fischer, M.E., *et al.* (1988) Cardiac rehabilitation after myocardial infarction: combined experience of randomised clinical trials. *Journal of the American Medical Association*, 260, 945–50.

Proudfoot, C., Thow, M., Rafferty, D. (2007) A UK survey of phase 1 cardiac rehabilitation for patients with acute coronary syndrome. *Physiotherapy*, 93(3), 183–8.

Royal College of Physicians London and the British Cardiac Society (RCP/BCS) (1975) Cardiac rehabilitation 1975. *Journal of the Royal College of Physicians London*, 9(4), 281–347.

Scottish Executive Health Department (2002) *Coronary Heart Disease and Stroke: Strategy for Scotland*. Edinburgh: Scottish Executive Health Department.

Scottish Intercollegiate Guidelines Network (SIGN) (2002) *SIGN Guideline No. 57: Cardiac Rehabilitation – A National Clinical Guideline*. Edinburgh: Scottish Intercollegiate Guidelines Network.

Service Framework for Cardiovascular Health and Wellbeing (SFCHW) (2008) *Belfast: Department of Health, Social Services and Public Safety*. Available from www.dhsspsni.gov.uk

Thow, M. (2006) *Exercise Leadership in Cardiac Rehabilitation: An Evidence Based Approach*. Chichester, UK: Wiley.

Thow, M., Hinton, S., Rafferty, D. (2006) *A Survey of Phase IV Cardiac Rehabilitation Provision in the UK*. BACR Conference, Warwickshire: Stratford Upon Avon.

Thow, M.K., Armstrong, G., Raffert, D. (2003) A survey to investigate the non-cardiac conditions and the physiotherapy interventions by physiotherapists in phase III cardiac rehabilitation exercise programmes. *Physiotherapy*, 89(4), 233–7.

2 Type 2 Diabetes

Alison Kirk and Lesley O'Brien

Chapter outline

Over the past years we have seen an increasing number of people with type 2 diabetes participating in programmes of cardiac rehabilitation (CR). This has occurred as a result of the increasing number of people being diagnosed with type 2 diabetes in association with increased levels of obesity. Furthermore, a large proportion of people with type 2 diabetes have cardiovascular disease. It is important therefore for health professionals working within CR to be aware of the current literature and guidelines surrounding exercise and type 2 diabetes. This chapter outlines the pathophysiology of diabetes, reviews current literature on the prevention and management of type 2 diabetes through physical activity and exercise, and provides guidelines on exercise prescription for this population. In addition, a short section on strategies to improve exercise adherence is included.

Pathophysiology and incidence of diabetes

Diabetes mellitus is a metabolic disorder characterised by chronic hyperglycaemia (raised blood glucose level) resulting from a deficiency of, and/or insensitivity to, the insulin hormone. Diabetes is suspected by the presence of symptoms such as excessive thirst and/or urination, unusual weight loss, extreme tiredness and blurred vision, and is diagnosed by measurements of abnormal blood glucose levels. In 1999 the World Health Organization (WHO) developed new diagnostic criteria for the range of blood glucose levels indicative of diabetes. These are as follows:
- Random venous plasma glucose ≥ 11.1 mmol/L or
- Fasting plasma glucose ≥ 7.0 mmol/L or
- Plasma glucose ≥ 11.1 mmol/L 2 hours after a 75-g oral glucose load (oral glucose tolerance test)

The new criteria include a decrease in fasting plasma glucose from 7.8 to 7.0 mmol/L. This change occurred as a result of new research associating poor glycaemic control with the development of diabetes complications (WHO, 1999).

Type 1 diabetes

Although there are a number of different types of diabetes, the two main forms are type 1 and type 2 diabetes. Type 1 diabetes, previously referred to as insulin-dependent diabetes mellitus, occurs as a result of an autoimmune response which is directed at the pancreas and causes the insulin-producing cells, known as beta cells, to be destroyed. The result is an absolute deficiency of insulin. Type 1 diabetes is less common than type 2 diabetes, accounting for approximately 10–16% of all people with diabetes. This condition develops most frequently in children and young adults and is generally diagnosed before the age of 30. The symptoms of type 1 diabetes develop rapidly and patients require insulin to survive. In addition to insulin therapy, leading a healthy lifestyle including healthy eating and adequate amounts of physical activity is important in type 1 and type 2 diabetes (ACSM, 2006).

Type 2 diabetes

Type 2 diabetes, previously referred to as non-insulin-dependent diabetes mellitus, involves a variable degree of defective insulin secretion as a result of beta-cell dysfunction and insulin resistance. The WHO defines insulin resistance as insulin sensitivity, under hyperinsulinemic euglycaemic clamp conditions (the gold standard for investigating and quantifying insulin resistance), below the lowest quartile for the population under investigation (WHO, 1999). This form of diabetes constitutes approximately 90–95% of all people with diabetes and is most commonly diagnosed in adults over the age of 40. Type 2 diabetes is increasingly appearing in children as a result of an increase in childhood obesity and/or decrease in physical activity (Diabetes UK, 2007). The symptoms of type 2 diabetes appear more gradually than the symptoms of type 1 diabetes and as a result a diagnosis may not be made for some years. It has been suggested that there may be as many people with undiagnosed type 2 diabetes as there are diagnosed cases. Thus, the number of people with type 2 diabetes in future could be massive and have serious consequences to the health care system. People with type 2 diabetes should be encouraged to lead a healthy lifestyle with healthy eating and adequate levels of physical activity (Diabetes UK, 2007). They may also need to take oral hypoglycaemic tablets (such as metformin, gliclazide or rosiglitazone) and/or insulin to control blood glucose levels.

Metabolic syndrome

People with type 2 diabetes often present with a clustering of risk factors for cardiovascular disease. These include dyslipidemia (specifically high triglycerides and low high-density lipoprotein cholesterol (HDL-C)), impaired glucose regulation and hyperinsulinaemia due to insulin resistance, obesity (including increased intra-abdominal adipose tissue), hypertension, impaired endothelial function and pro-coagulant state. This clustering of risk factors is often termed as the insulin resistance, syndrome X or metabolic syndrome (ACSM, 2006). Physical activity may be an especially attractive preventive or therapeutic intervention towards the metabolic syndrome since research has clearly identified that it can be beneficial for more than one (if not all) components of the metabolic syndrome (ACSM, 2006). In individuals with metabolic syndrome who undertake a programme of physical activity, it may be useful to monitor the different components of the metabolic syndrome to determine and provide feedback on the full spectrum of beneficial effects.

Incidence of diabetes

Amos and colleagues in 1997 projected global prevalence of diabetes for the years up to 2010 using published prevalence rates in addition to current and projected age distributions, survival rates and developments in economic status. In 1997, 124 million people were estimated to have diabetes, representing approximately 2.1% of world populations; 97% of this total had type 2 diabetes. The prevalence of diabetes is rapidly increasing, and it is estimated that a total of 221 million people worldwide will have diabetes by the year 2010 (Amos *et al.*, 1997). In 2004 in the UK, the population with diagnosed diabetes was 2.3 million with the vast majority suffering from type 2 diabetes, representing almost 4% of the population (Diabetes UK, 2007). The prevalence of type 2 diabetes increases rapidly with age and is higher in ethnic groups, being six times more common in people of South Asian descent and up to three times more common amongst those of African and African Caribbean origin (Amos *et al.*, 1997).

Financial cost of diabetes

Type 2 diabetes is a serious burden to health care resources. It is estimated that type 2 diabetes alone costs the UK National Health Service (NHS) £2 billion per year, approximately 4.7% of total NHS expenditure. An additional £36 million is estimated to be spent on related social services and private health care costs. The high cost is largely caused by treatment of complications of diabetes, which increases overall spending for an affected patient more than fivefold (Moore, 2000). The total expense is likely to be significantly underestimated as a result of the high number of undiagnosed cases and the misclassification of the cause of complications. The rising prevalence of type 2 diabetes and the associated drain on the NHS make this condition one of the most challenging health problems of the twenty-first century. Clearly, effective methods of managing type 2 diabetes and, in particular, preventing associated complications will substantially reduce the costs of this condition.

Complications of diabetes

Prolonged exposure to raised blood glucose levels damages tissues throughout the body. Microvascular complications, which are specific to diabetes, include diabetic retinopathy, leading to visual impairment and blindness, and diabetic nephropathy, leading to progressive renal failure and diabetic neuropathy. Neuropathy of the lower limbs can lead to loss of sensation in the feet, increasing the risk of foot ulcers and lower limb amputations. Damage to other nerves in the body can lead to a variety of further complications, including postural hypotension, abnormal sweating, gastrointestinal problems and erectile dysfunction.

In terms of microvascular complications, compared to people without diabetes, people with type 2 diabetes have a two- to fourfold higher risk of cardiovascular disease (Diabetes UK, 2007; Kannel and McGee, 1979). This is the leading cause of mortality in the population with diabetes, with up to 75% of deaths being due to cardiovascular disease. Haffner *et al.* (1998) reported that people with type 2 diabetes without prior myocardial infarction (MI) had as high a risk of a new MI as people without diabetes who already has had an MI. In view of the excessive cardiovascular disease in this population, diabetes had been described as 'a state of premature cardiovascular death' (Fisher and Shaw, 2001). Tuomilehto *et al.* (2001) reported that improvements in glycaemic control led to clear reductions in microvascular complication, but only borderline reductions in macrovascular complications. This highlights the importance of incorporating interventions in diabetes management designed to improve cardiovascular disease risk factors as well as interventions to improve glycaemic control. Exercise and physical activity are potentially such interventions. In 2002 the United Kingdom Prospective Diabetes Study Group (UKPDSG) treatment of hypertension was identified as being particularly important, having been shown to reduce both macrovascular and microvascular complications in subjects with diabetes (UKPDSG, 2002).

Diabetes and survival after myocardial infarction

A small number of studies have examined the effect of diabetes on short-term prognosis following first acute myocardial infarction (AMI). Most studies (Chun *et al.*, 1997; Lehto *et al.*, 1994; Mak *et al.*, 1997) have shown that patients with diabetes who have suffered a first AMI have a significantly higher mortality rate than myocardial patients without diabetes. A study by Melchior *et al.* (1996), however, failed to demonstrate this relationship. Mortality rates in post-MI patients with diabetes vary from 10.5 to 40% and are between 40 and 100% higher than post-MI patients without diabetes (Lehto *et al.*, 1994). Among people with diabetes, mortality rates over 30 days have been shown to be significantly higher in women compared to men (Chun *et al.*, 1997; Lehto *et al.*, 1994; Rosengren *et al.*, 2001) and in people treated with insulin compared to those treated with oral hypoglycaemic agents or with diet alone (Mak *et al.*, 1997).

A larger number of studies have examined the effect of diabetes on long-term prognosis following first AMI. These studies consistently show significantly higher mortality rates in people with diabetes compared to those without diabetes over periods of between 1 and 10 years post-MI. People with diabetes often have a greater number of risk factors for MI than people without diabetes, but the significantly higher mortality rates remain after adjustment for the presence of risk factors. Similar to short-term survival, long-term survival rates among people with diabetes are significantly higher in women compared to men (Lowel *et al.*, 2000; Malmberg *et al.*, 2000; Mukamal *et al.*, 2001; Rosengren *et al.*, 2001) and in people treated with insulin compared to those treated with oral hypoglycaemic agents or with diet alone (Chun *et al.*, 2002; Gustafsson *et al.*, 2000; Mak *et al.*, 1997). A common criticism of studies investigating prognosis after AMI in people with diabetes is a lack of distinction between type 1 and type 2 diabetes. Although both types of diabetes are often considered together, type 1 and type 2 diabetes are different conditions, with different pathologies, treatments and complications. The lack of distinction makes it unclear whether the poor prognosis reported in patients with diabetes applies to a similar extent to patients with type 1 and type 2 diabetes.

The mortality from MI has changed over the last 20 years. Chun *et al.* (2002) examined the mortality related to the year of onset of coronary event symptoms using data from the WHO and the Monitoring Trends and Determinants of Cardiovascular Disease project. A significant decrease in 28-day fatality was recorded in post-MI patients without diabetes, and they suggested that this change was probably related to improvements in treatment. In comparison, no apparent improvement was recorded in post-MI mortality in patients with diabetes.

In a retrospective, incidence cohort study, Donnan *et al.* (2002) studied the incidence of death and macrovascular complications after first MI in 2028 patients with type 2 diabetes. In comparison to patients without diabetes, patients with diabetes had higher rates of hospitalisation for re-infarction, heart failure, stroke, angina and coronary artery bypass graft at 2 years. However, only the incidence of heart failure reached significance. A higher rate of heart failure in post-MI patients with diabetes compared to patients without diabetes has been reported in several studies (Chun *et al.*, 2002; Donnan *et al.*, 2002; Gustafsson *et al.*, 2000; Lehto *et al.*, 1994; Mak *et al.*, 1997; Malmberg *et al.*, 2000; Mukamal *et al.*, 2001). Mak *et al.* (1997) also reported significantly higher rates of stroke, recurrent infarction, recurrent ischaemia, sustained hypotension, cardiogenic shock, atrial fibrillation, atrioventricular block and asystole at 30 days and 1 year among post-MI patients with diabetes compared to patients without diabetes.

Possible explanations presented in the literature for the reduced survival after MI in people with diabetes are the following: higher levels of autonomic dysfunction leading to fewer people experiencing chest pain during a cardiac event; differences in treatment plans; higher blood glucose levels; larger and more frequent anterior infarcts in people with diabetes and higher levels of cardiac failure.

Prevention of type 2 diabetes through changes in lifestyle

There is now increasing evidence that many aspects of type 2 diabetes can be improved and possibly prevented by regular, frequent physical activity. The Finnish Diabetes Prevention Study carried out by Tuomilehto *et al.* (2001) provides strong evidence that lifestyle changes in people with impaired glucose tolerance can prevent or delay the onset of type 2 diabetes. This study randomly assigned 522 men and women with impaired glucose tolerance to an intervention group which received an individualised diet and physical activity programme, compared to a control group who received standard care. Participants were followed for an average of 3.2 years. At 1-year follow-up the intervention group recorded significantly greater self-reported improvements in both diet and exercise. The intervention group also recorded significantly greater improvements at 1 year in the following clinical and metabolic variables: body weight, waist circumference, fasting plasma glucose concentration and plasma glucose and serum insulin concentration 2 hours after oral glucose tolerance test, HDL-C, triglycerides and blood pressure. These changes, with the exception of HDL-C, were maintained at 2-year follow-up. Analysis of progression to type 2 diabetes showed that the cumulative incidence of diabetes was 58% lower in the intervention group compared to the control group.

The results of the National Institute of Health's Diabetes Prevention Study in the US (Knowler *et al.*, 2002), which compared the effectiveness of metformin (an antidiabetic agent) with an intensive lifestyle intervention to delay or prevent type 2 diabetes, confirmed the results of the Finnish study (Tuomilehto *et al.*, 2001) only with greater power. Both these studies highlight the importance of changes in lifestyle in people with impaired glucose tolerance to prevent or delay type 2 diabetes.

Benefits of exercise for people with type 2 diabetes

Exercise and physical activity have important physiological and psychological benefits for all people but particularly for people with established type 2 diabetes. For this reason physical activity and exercise are important components of good diabetes management.

Acute effects of exercise

Glucose levels

The increased metabolic demands that accompany exercise require an increase in fuel mobilisation from storage sites and an increase in fuel oxidation in the working muscle. Fuel mobilisation and utilisation during exercise are controlled by a precise endocrine response. Generally during exercise, in normal healthy individuals arterial insulin levels reduce and levels of glucagon, cortisol, epinephrine and norepinephrine increase. This precise endocrine response ensures that arterial glucose levels change very little during exercise up to a moderate intensity.

A few studies have evaluated the acute metabolic response to exercise in people with type 2 diabetes. During mild-to-moderate exercise, most individuals with type 2 diabetes exhibit decreases in blood glucose levels, with the effect sometimes persisting into the post-exercise period (Glacca *et al.*, 1998; Larsen *et al.*, 1997; Minuk *et al.*, 1981; Thompson *et al.*, 2001). An early study by Minuk and colleagues in 1981 investigated the metabolic responses to exercise in seven obese people with type 2 diabetes, maintained on diet or sulphonylurea (an antidiabetic agent) therapy, compared to seven obese controls without diabetes. Exercise consisted of 45 minutes on a cycle ergometer at 60% of maximal aerobic power. In people with diabetes, blood glucose levels fell by approximately 50 mg/dL during the 45-minute exercise session, while in control subjects blood glucose levels did not change. In people with diabetes this lower level of glycaemia was maintained into the post-exercise period.

The reason blood glucose levels decrease during mild-to-moderate exercise remains controversial. Minuk *et al.* (1981) attributed the decrease to an inadequate exercise-associated increase in hepatic glucose production coupled with normal increase in muscle glucose utilisation. The reduced rise in glucose production is suggested to be due to the failure of insulin to fall during exercise, as it does in control subjects, and/or to the hepatic effects of hyperglycaemia present in people with type 2 diabetes (Minuk *et al.*, 1981). In more recent studies a greater increase in glucose utilisation and a decrease in plasma insulin levels have been described (Larsen *et al.*, 1997).

In contrast to moderate-intensity exercise, short-term, high-intensity exercise has been shown to increase blood glucose levels during and for up to 1 hour after exercise. This rise in blood glucose has been associated with an exaggerated counter-regulatory hormone response. Kjaer *et al.* (1990) studied the effects of maximal exercise on glucoregulation in seven people with type 2 diabetes and seven healthy controls. The exercise protocol involved cycling at 60% of maximum aerobic power for 7 minutes, followed by 3 minutes at 100% of maximum aerobic power, and a further 2 minutes at 110% of maximum aerobic power. In subjects with type 2 diabetes, plasma glucose concentrations increased and remained elevated for 1-hour post-exercise. Plasma glucose concentrations in control subjects did not change significantly during exercise.

Insulin resistance

Insulin resistance is a major feature of type 2 diabetes. Regular exercise can improve insulin sensitivity and help to diminish elevated glucose levels towards normal (American Diabetes Association, 2001). Several studies have demonstrated that acute exercise increases insulin sensitivity. An early study by Devlin *et al.* (1987) demonstrated that a single session of high-intensity exercise at 85% of maximum aerobic power significantly increased peripheral and splanchnic insulin sensitivity, persisting for 12–16 hours post-exercise in a group of men with type 2 diabetes.

There is no consensus regarding the optimal intensity and duration of exercise required to improve insulin sensitivity. It has been shown that improvements in insulin sensitivity after walking at a high intensity (75% of maximum aerobic power) for a short duration and at a moderate intensity (50% of maximum aerobic power) with a longer duration were nearly identical and significantly higher than for sedentary controls (Braun *et al.*, 1995). The beneficial effects of light-intensity activity on insulin sensitivity have also been demonstrated. Usui *et al.* (1998) showed that an acute 30-minute session of light-intensity (40–50% of maximal aerobic power) cycling in obese people with type 2 diabetes improved insulin sensitivity.

The effect of an acute bout of exercise on insulin action is lost within a few days. Heath *et al.* (1983) illustrated that trained individuals lose much of their enhanced sensitivity to insulin within a few days of exercise termination. However, a single bout of exercise restores insulin sensitivity to the same level as in the trained state.

Current research suggests that frequent exercise performed at a low-to-moderate intensity is required to facilitate glucose reductions and improve insulin sensitivity in people with type 2 diabetes. However, most studies investigating the effects of acute exercise on glucose levels and insulin resistance in people with type 2 diabetes have used relatively small study groups, controlled by diet or oral antidiabetic therapy. Further research with larger and more diverse populations with diabetes is required in order to fully understand the effects of acute exercise in people with type 2 diabetes.

Long-term effects of exercise

Metabolic control

Regular, frequent physical activity holds important benefits for people with type 2 diabetes. A summary of potential benefits is illustrated in Box 2.1.

Box 2.1 Potential benefits of frequent physical activity in type 2 diabetes

- Improve glycaemic control
  - Blood glucose levels
  - Insulin resistance
- Improve cardiovascular risk profile
  - Lipid profile
  - Blood pressure
  - Cardiorespiratory fitness
  - Body composition
- Enhance quality of life and psychological status

Glycosylated haemoglobin (HbA_{1c}) is a measure of the amount of glucose attached to haemoglobin. The more the glucose in the blood, the higher the HbA_{1c} level. Haemoglobin has a lifespan of 2–3 months; therefore, HbA_{1c} gives a measure of blood glucose level averaged over the previous 2–3 months. A normal person without diabetes has an HbA_{1c} level of 3.5–5.5%. For people with diabetes SIGN (2001) recommends that an HbA_{1c} level of $\leq 7\%$ is considered good glycaemic control and highlights that long-term poor glycaemic control ($HbA_{1c} > 10\%$) is associated with increased risk of microvascular complications. Several studies have reported favourable changes in HbA_{1c} after physical activity training of variable type, duration and intensity (Honkola *et al.*, 1997; Raz *et al.*, 1994; Trovati *et al.*, 1984; Walker *et al.*, 1999). The favourable effect of frequent exercise on the requirements for hypoglycaemic medication has also been documented (Fujinuma *et al.*, 1999; Kevorkian, 1986). Fujinuma *et al.* (1999) investigated the effect of 3–4 weeks of supervised exercise in 78 people with type 2 diabetes. Compared to a control group of non-exercisers, a significantly greater number of participants in the exercise group discontinued or reduced their insulin dose. Of the 56 people allocated to the exercise group, 10 participants discontinued insulin injections and 36 reduced the number of insulin injections per day.

The majority of research investigating the effect of exercise in the management of type 2 diabetes has incorporated structured, supervised exercise programmes. A study by Walker *et al.* (1999) demonstrated that with correct education and encouragement an unsupervised exercise programme could also be carried out successfully. Participants in this study were 11 women with type 2 diabetes and 20 controls without diabetes. All participants were encouraged to walk for 1 hour on 5 days/week for 12 weeks. At 12-week follow-up significant improvements in body mass index, body fat, HbA_{1c}, total cholesterol and low-density lipoprotein cholesterol (LDL-C) were recorded. This study is limited, however, by a lack of randomisation.

Favourable changes in glucose control usually deteriorate within 72 hours of the last exercise session in people with type 2 diabetes (Devlin *et al.*, 1987). There is now a general consensus that improved glycaemic control over prolonged periods of frequent exercise participation is largely due to the cumulative effects of individual exercise bouts, as opposed to the long-term adaptations to physical activity training (Devlin *et al.*, 1987; Heath *et al.*, 1983). As a result, people with type 2 diabetes should participate in frequent exercise in order to sustain the glucose-lowering effects of exercise.

Not all studies have reported improvements in glycaemic control in response to exercise. Skarfors *et al.* (1987) studied the long-term effects of exercise training in a group of men over 60 years with type 2 diabetes. Exercise training incorporated supervised exercise sessions, twice weekly at 75% of maximal aerobic power for 45 minutes. At 2-year follow-up significant improvements in maximal aerobic power were demonstrated. However, no accompanying beneficial effects were shown in metabolic variables when compared to controls. Similar findings have been reported by Ligtenberg *et al.* (1997). In a randomised controlled trial the effects of exercise were investigated in a group of 92 obese, elderly (over 55 years) people with poorly controlled, advanced type 2 diabetes. The exercise intervention included individual, supervised exercise at an intensity of 60–80% of maximal aerobic power for 50 minutes, three times a week for 6 weeks. For a further 20 weeks, participants exercised at home, with encouragement being given for 6 weeks after the end of supervised exercise. At 6-week and 6-month follow-ups, significant between-group differences were recorded in self-reported physical activity levels and maximal aerobic power. No changes were observed in glucose tolerance or insulin sensitivity at any point during the study.

The results of these studies could suggest that exercise is more effective for improving glycaemic control during earlier stages of diabetes. Consistent with this suggestion, Barnard *et al.* (1994) demonstrated that the effect of exercise and diet on glycaemic control is related to treatment of diabetes, the effect of diet and exercise interventions being greatest in those participants receiving no medication or oral hypoglycaemic agents compared with participants taking insulin. These results stress the need for an early emphasis on lifestyle modification in the management of people with type 2 diabetes.

A meta-analysis (Boulé *et al.*, 2001) of 14 controlled clinical trials investigated the effect of either aerobic exercise training (12 studies) or resistance exercise training (2 studies) for at least 3 months' duration on HbA_{1c}. In comparison to non-intervention groups, exercise intervention groups significantly improved HbA_{1c} by 0.66%. This is a clinically significant improvement, which, if maintained, could substantially reduce the risk and progression of diabetes complications.

Cardiovascular benefit

Regular exercise and physical activity have been associated with reduced cardiovascular and all-cause mortality in people with type 2 diabetes. In a prospective cohort study, Gregg *et al.* (2003) compared inactive people with diabetes to those with diabetes who walked at least 2 hours/week. In this comparison study those who walked at least 2 hours/week had a 39% lower all-cause mortality rate and a 34% lower cardiovascular disease mortality rate. These results were controlled for sex, age, race, body mass index, smoking and presence of comorbid conditions. The mortality rates were lowest for persons who walked 3–4 hours/week (54% reduction) and for those who reported that their walking involved moderate increases in heart and breathing rates (43% reduction). The protective association of physical activity was observed for persons of varying sex, age, race, body mass index, diabetes duration, comorbid conditions and physical limitations.

Exercise has also been associated with improvements in cardiovascular risk profile in people with type 2 diabetes. Research has shown that after exercise training individuals with type 2 diabetes experience favourable changes in lipid profile, including reduced total cholesterol (Ligtenberg *et al.*, 1997; Walker *et al.*, 1999), reduced triglycerides (Honkola *et al.*, 1997; Lehmann *et al.*, 1995; Raz *et al.*, 1994; Taniguchi *et al.*, 2000), increased HDL-C (Lehmann *et al.*, 1995) and reduced LDL-C (Honkola *et al.*, 1997; Walker *et al.*, 1999), reduced blood pressure (Lehmann *et al.*, 1995), improved cardiorespiratory fitness (Aliev *et al.*, 1993; Brandenburg *et al.*, 1999; Mourier *et al.*, 1997) and improved psychological well-being (Ligtenberg *et al.*, 1998). These beneficial effects of exercise on cardiovascular risk are especially important in light of the increased independent risk of cardiovascular disease in this population.

Lehmann *et al.* (1995) investigated the effect of an individualised, moderate-intensity aerobic exercise programme in people with type 2 diabetes. Exercise was performed under supervision once weekly and participants were encouraged, through goal setting, self-monitoring and social support, to include a further three unsupervised exercise sessions a week. At 3-month follow-up participants in the experimental group recorded significant improvements compared to controls in physical activity levels, blood pressure, waist-to-hip ratio and plasma lipids, with a 20% reduction in triglyceride and an increase in HDL subfractions. There were no changes in glycaemic control (HbA$_{1c}$) in the experimental group. However, the control group increased glycaemia control on average by 0.6%.

The effect of resistance training on cardiovascular risk has been demonstrated. Honkola *et al.* (1997) evaluated the effects of an individualised, progressive resistance training programme on blood pressure, lipid profile and glycaemic control in people with type 2 diabetes. A moderate-intensity, high-volume, low-resistance supervised resistance training programme was carried out twice weekly for 5 months. At 5-month follow-up the experimental group, in comparison to the control group, recorded significant improvements in total cholesterol, LDL-C and triglycerides. Body weight and glycaemic control did not change significantly in the experimental group, but increased in the control group. The difference between groups in the change in body weight and glycaemic control achieved statistical significance. No significant changes were recorded in blood pressure for either group. This study could, however, be criticised for a lack of randomisation, and as a result the majority of men participated in the experimental group and women in the control group. These studies illustrate the benefits of exercise on cardiovascular risk factors but only incorporate a relatively short-term follow-up period. Further evidence is needed to confirm that the benefits observed can be maintained over a longer period (Thompson *et al.*, 2001).

Low cardiorespiratory fitness has been directly associated with cardiovascular disease and all-cause mortality in the general population (Blair *et al.*, 1996). In a recent prospective cohort study, similar findings were reported in people with type 2 diabetes. Ming *et al.* (2000) observed 1263 men (50 ± 10 years of age) with type 2 diabetes and mortality documented for an average of 12 years. After adjustment for age, baseline cardiovascular disease, fasting plasma glucose level, high cholesterol, overweight, smoking status, high blood pressure and family history of cardiovascular disease, men with low cardiorespiratory fitness had an adjusted relative risk for all-cause mortality of 2.1 compared with fit men. Kohl *et al.* (1992) demonstrated a similar inverse relationship between cardiorespiratory fitness and mortality in people with variable levels of glycaemic control. Although risk of death increases with higher glycaemic status, the adverse impact of hyperglycaemia on mortality appears to be reduced with increased fitness.

Maximal aerobic power (VO_2max) is the gold standard measure of overall cardiorespiratory fitness and describes the highest oxygen uptake obtainable by an individual for a given form of exercise. Several studies have demonstrated that people with type 2 diabetes have a reduced oxygen consumption at submaximal (Katoh *et al.*, 1996; Vanninen *et al.*, 1992) and maximal exercise when compared with healthy age-matched controls (Katoh *et al.*, 1996; Regensteiner *et al.*, 1994, 1998).

The causes of this impaired exercise capacity are unknown. Research has shown a strong inverse association between cardiorespiratory fitness and development of type 2 diabetes (Vanninen *et al.*, 1992). This raises the possibility that reduced cardiorespiratory fitness may contribute to the development of type 2 diabetes and could potentially serve as a marker for individuals at high risk. There is also evidence to suggest that both central (cardiac) (Regensteiner *et al.*, 1998; Roy *et al.*, 1989; Wei *et al.*, 1999) and peripheral factors (Liang *et al.*, 1997; Simoneau and Kelley, 1997) may relate to the impaired exercise capacity associated with type 2 diabetes.

Several studies have reported improvements in VO_2max as a result of exercise training in people with type 2 diabetes (Aliev *et al.*, 1993; Brandenburg *et al.*, 1999; Ligtenberg *et al.*, 1997; Mourier *et al.*, 1997). Ligtenberg *et al.* (1997) found significant improvements in VO_2max in elderly people with type 2 diabetes after 6 weeks of moderate-intensity supervised exercise.

After 15 weeks of individualised exercise at 40–60% of VO_2max, Khan and Rupp (1995) also reported significant improvements in VO_2max.

Psychological benefit of exercise

While the psychological effects of exercise have been studied to a great extent in the general population, a few studies have investigated the association between physical activity and psychological well-being in people with diabetes. Stewart *et al.* (1994) in a 2-year observational study showed higher levels of physical activity to be associated with overall better psychological functioning and well-being in people with either type 1 or type 2 diabetes. Glasgow *et al.* (1997) investigated the association between quality of life and demographic, medical history and self-management characteristics of people with diabetes. Quality of life was assessed using the physical functioning, social functioning and mental health scales of the Medical Outcomes Study SF-20 questionnaire. A total of 2800 people with type 1 and type 2 diabetes were sent questionnaires. A response rate of 73.4% was obtained. Findings from the study revealed physical activity participation to be the only significant self-management behaviour predictive of enhanced quality of life.

In a more randomised controlled trial, Ligtenberg *et al.* (1998) assessed the influence of an exercise training programme on psychological well-being in 51 elderly people with type 2 diabetes. After 6 weeks of supervised training for three 1-hour sessions per week, at 60–80% of VO_2max, significant improvements were found in both VO_2max and all subscales of the well-being questionnaire, except depression. At the end of the supervised exercise period, participants were advised to continue training at home without supervision. A follow-up was conducted 14 weeks after the supervised exercise period ended. At this follow-up, although VO_2max remained significantly higher than in the control group, well-being scores had returned to baseline level. These results could suggest that social support achieved during supervised group exercise is an important factor for the enhanced psychological well-being apparent after exercise training. The development of social support through family or friends should therefore receive high priority when developing individualised unsupervised exercise programmes for people with type 2 diabetes.

Physical activity habits in type 2 diabetes

Physical activity participation

Despite the reported potential benefits of exercise, it has been suggested that 60–80% of people with type 2 diabetes remain inactive, possibly related to large percentage of people with type 2 diabetes being overweight (Ford and Herman, 1995; Hays and Clark, 1999; Krug *et al.*, 1991). While people with diabetes report exercise rates similar to those of the general population, people with diabetes report a significantly greater frequency of exercise relapse (Krug et al., 1991). Furthermore, the greatest number of people with diabetes report low adherence to exercise recommendations compared to other diabetes self-care behaviours (Ford and Herman, 1995).

Participation of patients with diabetes in CR

The effectiveness of CR programmes in people with diabetes has been examined in a small number of studies (Lucas et al., 2000; Milani and Lavie, 1996; Suresh et al., 2001; Verges et al., 2001). Suresh et al. (2001) investigated clinical outcomes and lifestyle modification at 1 year in people with diabetes attending a standard CR programme following MI. The CR programme incorporated dietetic, physiotherapy (exercise) and psychology services and was coordinated by CR nurses. The programme included exercise classes implemented 6 weeks after an AMI. These classes lasted 1 hour and were held twice a week for 6 weeks, and then once a week indefinitely. Patients were also invited to attend weekly sessions on relaxation and stress management. Patient's progress was monitored at 3, 6 and 12 months. At 1-year follow-up, compared to post-MI patients without diabetes, patients with diabetes were less likely to be on aspirin (75% vs 90%, $p < 0.01$) or β-blockers (39% vs 61%, $p < 0.001$), achieve at least 6 minutes during an exercise tolerance test (37% vs 49%, $p = 0.03$), attend the exercise class (27% vs 59%, $p < 0.001$) and have stopped smoking (54% vs 69%, $p = 0.003$). At 1-year follow-up both all-cause and cardiovascular mortalities were significantly higher in people with diabetes compared to those without (all-cause: people with diabetes – 15.7% vs people without diabetes – 5.6%, $p < 0.001$; cardiac: people with diabetes – 13.4% vs people without diabetes – 5.4%, $p < 0.001$). The authors concluded that a standard programme of CR following AMI was less effective for patients with diabetes than for those without. They suggested that patients with diabetes required specialised programmes of rehabilitation in order to integrate the care of diabetes with their recent AMI.

In a similar study, Milani and Lavie (1996) compared the effectiveness of a standard 12-week CR programme in people with diabetes and people without diabetes after AMI. At 12-week follow-up, people without diabetes had significant improvements in lipid profile, body weight, percentage body fat, exercise capacity and several parameters of quality of life. In comparison to patients with diabetes, apart from an improvement in exercise capacity, no other improvements in physiological parameters were achieved. Parameters of quality of life improved by a similar extent to that seen in the people without diabetes. Unfortunately, no information is given on adherence to the different components of the CR programme.

Two further studies (Lucas et al., 2000; Verges et al., 2001), which examined the effectiveness of a programme of CR for people with diabetes, reported significantly smaller improvements in exercise capacity (peak

VO_2 mL/kg/min and workload achieved) in patients with diabetes compared to those without. Possible contributors to the lack of improvement in exercise capacity revealed that HbA_{1c} is the only significant confounding factor in these studies.

Variables associated with physical activity participation of patients with diabetes

Limited research has examined variables associated with physical activity participation in people with diabetes. Hays and Clark (1999) reported higher education level and younger age as significant correlates of physical activity participation in people with type 2 diabetes. In contrast, Krug et al. (1991) reported that older people with type 2 diabetes were more likely to exercise than younger people. Swift et al. (1995) found older age and greater time since diagnosis was associated with the length of time subjects maintained regular physical activity. These findings could be related to the health belief model (Rosenstock, 1974). This model proposes that adherence to a health behaviour depends on the perceived severity of illness threat, perceptions of vulnerability to illness if no action is taken and the belief that the effectiveness of the behaviour outweighs barriers to making the change. Increasing age and duration of diabetes, with the onset of diabetes complications, may influence perceived susceptibility and severity of diabetes and may explain why people with type 2 diabetes delay initiating an exercise programme until a later age.

Among the cognitive variables, self-efficacy (a person's confidence in his or her ability to carry out a behaviour) has been identified as an important predictor of exercise participation in people with type 2 diabetes. Kingery and Glasgow (1989) examined the relationship of self-efficacy in predicting diabetes self-care behaviours, including diet, exercise and glucose testing in people with type 2 diabetes. Exercise self-efficacy proved to be a moderately strong predictor of exercise participation. However, of the three self-care behaviours, participants rated themselves lowest on exercise self-efficacy. These findings are consistent with a study conducted by Padgett (1991) and highlight the importance of physical activity interventions designed to enhance self-efficacy for improving exercise adherence in people with type 2 diabetes. Other cognitive variables that have been shown to be associated with exercise participation in people with type 2 diabetes include perceived benefits and barriers to physical activity participation (Wilson et al., 1986), performance and outcome expectations (Kingery and Glasgow, 1989), motivation and physical activity knowledge (Hays and Clark, 1999).

Wilson et al. (1986) reported that people with type 2 diabetes believe in the effectiveness of medication treatments of diabetes, but report the lowest amount of belief in the effectiveness of exercise. This highlights the need to explain the rationale behind the effectiveness of exercise in the management of type 2 diabetes. Perceived benefits of exercise for people with type 2 diabetes include improving diabetes control and managing weight (Swift *et al.*, 1995). Reported barriers include physical discomfort from exercise, fears of reactions from low blood sugars, being too overweight to exercise and lack of social support (Swift *et al.*, 1995; Wilson *et al.*, 1986). Identification of perceived barriers to physical activity participation and education on how to overcome them, that is monitoring of blood glucose, could significantly reduce reported barriers and therefore enhance adherence to physical activity.

Low motivation to participate in physical activity is a major factor associated with poor physical activity participation and dropout in healthy individuals (Dishman and Ickes, 1981). Hays and Clark (1999) reported motivation for physical activity to be significantly associated with physical activity participation in people with type 2 diabetes. These findings suggest that effective methods for enhancing motivation should be included in the promotion of physical activity in people with type 2 diabetes. Goal-setting and self-monitoring of progress are important sources of self-motivation (see Thow, 2006, Ch. 8). Martin *et al.* (1984) found that flexible exercise goals set by the individual, in comparison to instructor set goals, significantly improved adherence to an exercise programme and to long-term maintenance of physical activity following completion of the programme.

Physical activity knowledge has been shown to correlate poorly with physical activity behaviour in the general population (King *et al.*, 1992). Similar findings have been reported in people with diabetes (Guion *et al.*, 2000). Guion *et al.* (2000) assessed knowledge of exercise in people with type 2 diabetes. Questionnaire results revealed that only 38% of respondents knew the recommended amounts of exercise. Consistent with previous research, a weak relationship was present between knowing recommended exercise amounts and actual reported physical activity participation. Similar findings have been reported from other health behaviours, suggesting that awareness of desired health practices is not sufficient for bringing about the adoption of health behaviour change.

Social support has been consistently correlated with physical activity participation in the general population (Wankel, 1984). People with type 2 diabetes report the lowest level of social support for exercise compared to other self-care behaviours (Wilson *et al.*, 1986). Furthermore, lack of social support is one of the most frequently cited barriers to exercise participation among people with type 2 diabetes (Swift *et al.*, 1995). These findings are highlighted by data reporting that although 76% of people with type 2 diabetes are advised to exercise regularly, only 21% receive instructions about the most beneficial type and amount of exercise. In comparison, 76% of people with type 2 diabetes receive dietary instructions (Ary *et al.*, 1986). A study by Marsden (1996) reported that people with type 1 diabetes perceived a poor service for exercise from health professionals, indicating that they did not receive adequate exercise education, support or encouragement.

Physical activity prescription

Physical activity prescription in the general population

Guidelines from the American College of Sports Medicine (ACSM) for exercise prescription result from research about the quality and quantity of exercise required to develop and maintain cardiorespiratory fitness. These guidelines recommend 20–60 minutes of moderate- to high-intensity endurance exercise (60–90% of maximum heart rate or 50–85% of maximum aerobic power) performed 3–5 days a week (ACSM, 1990).

More recently, the ACSM has suggested 20–60 minutes of continuous or accumulated (e.g. accumulated 10-minute bouts six times per day) exercise. The level of exercise should be 60–80% of heart rate reserve (HHR) or 77–90% maximum heart rate (MHR) equivalent to 12–16 rating of perceived exertion (RPR) (ACSM, 2006; Borg, 1982).

Physical activity prescription in people with type 2 diabetes

Changes in cardiovascular health do not necessarily parallel improvements in cardiorespiratory fitness. A review of physiological, epidemiological and clinical evidence outlined that participation in moderate-intensity physical activity, which did not exert an effect on cardiorespiratory fitness, had potential to improve health. In view of this new research, the American College of Sports Medicine and Centers of Disease Control and Prevention developed additional exercise guidelines focusing on improving health (Pate *et al.*, 1995). These guidelines recommend accumulating 30 minutes of moderate-intensity physical activity (60–79% of MHR or 50–74% of maximum aerobic power) on most days of the week. These guidelines appear more acceptable to the whole population where the lower levels of intensity are less threatening and tolerated better. A study assessing participation in exercise found that in an obese population the exercise intensity at lower levels of 60–70% of MHR was achieved by twice as many of the obese participants (34%) as the traditional recommendations (17%) (Weyer *et al.*, 1998). For the general, more active population, exercising can be at the higher end of the intensity guidelines; for diabetic and overweight groups, intensity should be set at the lower end of the spectrum where health benefits may be accrued and adherence improved.

Cardiorespiratory prescription

The ACSM published a position statement outlining exercise prescription for people with type 2 diabetes (ACSM, 2000, 2006). These guidelines recommend that people with type 2 diabetes, with no significant complications or limitations, should aim to achieve a minimum cumulative total of 1000 kcal/week in aerobic activity in order to achieve health-related benefits (ACSM, 2006). The addition of a well-balanced resistance training programme will further improve and maintain muscular strength and body composition. In addition, to achieve weight loss people with type 2 diabetes should aim for up to ≤2000 kcal/week. The exercise can be achieved via participation in structured exercise or through accumulate daily exercise, for example walking and stair climbing (ACSM, 2006).

In view of research demonstrating that favourable changes in glucose tolerance and insulin sensitivity deteriorate within 72 hours of physical activity participation, frequent physical activity participation is important for people with type 2 diabetes. Frequency of physical activity should be at least 3–4 days/week. Furthermore, a low-to-moderate intensity of physical activity, 50–80% (oxygen uptake reserve) VO_2R or HRR (Karvonen *et al.*, 1957), is recommended in order to achieve these metabolic improvements (ACSM, 2006). The intensity of activity should be at comfortable level of exertion in order to minimise risk and maximise health benefits and, most importantly, enhance the likelihood of adherence to the physical activity programme. The rate of perceived exertion (RPE) should be 11–14 (Borg, 1982) (see Thow, 2006, pp. 68–81, for application of RPE). Exercise should be performed for a cumulative duration of 20–60 minutes (ACSM, 2006). Similarly, when weight loss is the primary goal, the duration should be incrementally increased to 60 minutes (Wallace, 1997). In addition, people with diabetes should aim to adopt an active living approach, for example using stairs rather than escalator and walking rather than driving (Blair and Church, 2004).

If no complications to exercise exist, the mode of exercise a person with diabetes performs is a matter of personal preference. The majority of the research documenting the benefits of exercise for people with diabetes involves aerobic activity, using large muscle groups, such as walking, cycling, aerobics and rowing. Many patients with type 2 diabetes are overweight and/or obese. (For more guidance on exercise for these patients, see Thow, 2006, pp. 123–5.)

Resistance training

Resistance training exercise has been shown to improve glucose utilisation and plasma lipid profile, associated with increasing muscle mass (Eriksson *et al.*, 1997; Ishii *et al.*, 1998). Resistance training should be carried out for a minimum of two sessions per week (48 hours between sessions). The intensity should be of a lower resistance (between 40 and 60% of one RM) and comprise one to three sets of 10–15 repetitions, progressing to 15–20 repetitions, and involve eight to ten different exercises for each major muscle group (ACSM, 2006).

For previously sedentary people with no history of exercise participation, an initial low-intensity exercise programme is recommended, with a gradual progressive increase in workload. To prevent musculoskeletal

Table 2.1 Exercise recommendations for people with diabetes with no complication.

Component of training	Frequency (sessions per week)	Intensity	Duration	Activity
Cardiorespiratory	3–4 days/week Adopt healthy living activity	50–80% VO$_2$R or HHR; RPE 11–14	20–60 minutes	Dynamic activity of large muscles
Resistance	Two sessions per week (48 hours between sessions)	40–60% one RM (avoid MMF)	1–3 sets, 10–15 repetitions progress to 15–20	8–10 different exercises for major muscle groups
Caloric expenditure	Accumulate per week			1000 kcal/week (2000 kcal/week weight loss)

Adapted from ACSM (2006, p. 208), Franklin and Gordon (2005, p. 335) and Blair and Church (2004).

VO$_2$R, oxygen uptake reserve; HHR, heart rate reserve; RPE, rate of perceived exertion; RM, repetition max; MMF, momentary muscle fatigue.

injuries a proper warm-up of at least 10–15 minutes and cool-down period of 10 minutes should be included prior to and at the end of the exercise session (Thow, 2006). See Table 2.1 for exercise recommendations for people with diabetes with no other complications.

Exercise prescription for people with diabetic complications

An area of ongoing concern is the possible adverse effect of physical activity on existing complications of diabetes. People with diabetes complications are often told to refrain from exercise for fear of deterioration of the condition and development of further complications. This leads to further compromise of physical and cardiovascular conditioning. It is important to develop exercise prescriptions for individuals with diabetes complications that will result in improved participation in normal activities and psychosocial well-being, whilst minimising the risk of further deterioration. A summary of diabetic complications and physical activity recommendations is displayed in Table 2.2.

Retinopathy
In theory, physical activity and exercise could have a potential detrimental effect on diabetic retinopathy by raising systolic blood pressure. However, at present there is no evidence of an association between physical activity participation and development or progression of diabetic retinopathy. In the Wisconsin epidemiological study of diabetic retinopathy (Cruickshanks *et al.*, 1992), higher levels of physical activity in women

Table 2.2 Diabetic complications and physical activity recommendations.

Diabetic complication	Physical activity recommendation
Retinopathy	Recommend walking, swimming, cycling. Avoid strenuous, Valsalva-type or jarring exercise.
Peripheral artery disease	Recommend interval training swimming, stationary cycling, chair exercises. Nudging leg pain.
Peripheral neuropathy	Recommend non-weight-bearing exercise (cycling, rowing, swimming). Avoid heavy weight-bearing exercise (running, prolonged walking, step exercise). Emphasis on foot and hand care. Avoid exercise causing rapid body position, heart rate or blood pressure changes.
Autonomic neuropathy	Recommend water exercise, semi-recumbent cycling. Avoid exercise causing rapid body position, heart rate or blood pressure changes.
Nephropathy	Recommend light-to-moderate exercise.

were associated with a reduced risk of proliferative diabetic retinopathy. No association was found in men. The possibility that people with multiple diabetic complications could be less likely to participate in exercise should not be overlooked. Bernbaum *et al.* (1989) assessed the effects of a 12-week moderate-intensity exercise programme in subjects with multiple diabetes complications including retinopathy. No deterioration of retinopathy was reported, and significant improvements were recorded in exercise tolerance, glycaemic control and insulin requirements.

Activities such as walking, swimming, low-impact aerobics and cycling are encouraged for people with retinopathy. Strenuous anaerobic exercise, exercise involving Valsalva-type manoeuvres or jarring movements and activities that lower the head below the waist may be contraindicated (Graham and McCarthey, 1990).

Peripheral artery disease

Research evaluating the effects of physical activity on peripheral artery disease (PAD) and intermittent claudication (IC) in people with diabetes is limited. A number of studies evaluating the effects of physical activity for people without diabetes with PAD have reported improvements in symptoms. Hiatt *et al.* (1989) demonstrated in a randomised controlled trial that 12 weeks of exercise training for people with PAD improved peak exercise performance, delayed the onset and progression of claudication pain during exercise and improved walking ability. Interval circuit training swimming, stationary cycling and chair exercises are all recommended activities for people with PAD (Graham and McCarthey, 1990; SIGN, 2006) (see Chapter 6 for more on PVD and IC).

Peripheral neuropathy

Limited research has evaluated the effects of physical activity on people with peripheral neuropathy. Complications of peripheral neuropathy, with the development of the foot abnormalities such as insensate foot, indicate that weight-bearing exercise, particularly prolonged walking, running or step exercise, should be undertaken with care or avoided. The repetitive stress and pressure from these types of exercise can lead to ulceration and fractures.

To minimise the risk of injury, non-weight-bearing exercise, such as cycling, rowing, swimming and chair exercises, should be encouraged. For people with neuropathy performing weight-bearing exercise, emphasis on foot care and decreasing foot pressure by wearing proper footwear is essential (Graham and McCarthey, 1990).

Autonomic neuropathy

Autonomic neuropathy is associated with reduced aerobic capacity (Hilstead *et al.*, 1979) and an increase in risk of an adverse cardiovascular event or sudden death during exercise (Kahn *et al.*, 1986). Hilstead *et al.* (1979) demonstrated a reduced maximal oxygen uptake, accompanied by an impaired heart rate response, from exercise in people with autonomic neuropathy, in comparison to those with no autonomic neuropathy. Impaired heart rate response makes the use of heart rate to measure exercise intensity inappropriate for people with autonomic neuropathy. Instead, subjective perceptions of intensity using, for example, the RPE scale should be used (Borg, 1982).

Blood pressure response during exercise, and with changes in posture, may be abnormal and ventilatory reflexes impaired in people with autonomic neuropathy. Tantucci *et al.* (1996) found that people with diabetic autonomic neuropathy, in comparison to both people with diabetes and those with no autonomic neuropathy and healthy controls, had an increased respiratory rate and alveolar ventilation in response to submaximal incremental exercise.

Activities that cause rapid changes in body position, heart rate or blood pressure should be avoided. Water exercises and semi-recumbent cycling are recommended for those with orthostatic hypotension, since the semi-recumbent posture and the pressure of water surrounding the body help to maintain blood pressure (Albright, 1998). The ability to recognise symptoms of hypoglycaemia is often reduced or absent in people with autonomic neuropathy. Awareness of hypoglycaemia and of blood glucose monitoring before, often during and after exercise can help to protect against episodes of hypoglycaemia. In addition, thermoregulation may be impaired. Loss of sweating function may cause dry, brittle skin and contribute to ulcer formation. Proper foot care and adequate hydration should be encouraged, and exercise in extreme temperatures avoided.

Nephropathy

During and immediately after acute exercise, albuminuria excretion rate increases. This effect has been associated with the rise in systolic blood pressure during exercise (Dahlquist *et al.*, 1983). No evidence is available to suggest that this acute effect leads to renal impairment in the long term. With a cohort of 372 people with type 2 diabetes, Calle-Pascual *et al.* (2001) evaluated the effect of regular physical activity on the appearance of microalbuminuria. Results revealed that the presence of normoalbuminuria is related to the level of physical activity, when corrected for blood pressure, duration of diabetes and glycaemic control. The higher the physical activity level, the higher the prevalence of normoalbuminuria.

At present, it is generally recommended that people with nephropathy should avoid high-intensity strenuous physical activity (Mogensen, 1995), but light- to moderate-intensity activity is safe and should be encouraged in this patient group.

Pre-exercise evaluation

Most people, including those with diabetes, can undertake exercise with a high level of safety. Exercise, however, is not without risk, and the recommendation that people with diabetes participate in an exercise programme is on the basis that the benefits outweigh the risks. To minimise possible risks when developing an exercise prescription, particular attention should be paid to appropriate screening, programme design, monitoring and patient education. The American Diabetes Association (ADA), in collaboration with the ACSM, published a position statement to further current understanding about the role of exercise in people with type 1 and type 2 diabetes (ADA, 2001).

Clinical assessment

Prior to participation in an exercise programme, the ADA (2001) and ACSM (2000) recommend that people with diabetes have a medical evaluation in order to screen for the presence of micro- and macrovascular complications that could potentially deteriorate as a result of participation in exercise. Identification of existing complications will assist in the development of an individualised exercise prescription with minimal risk to the patient.

Exercise test

The ADA (2001) and ACSM (2000) also recommend an exercise tolerance test prior to participation in moderate- to high-intensity exercise if a person with diabetes is at a high risk for underlying cardiovascular disease, based on one of the following criteria:
- Age >35 years
- Type 2 diabetes of >10 years' duration
- Type 1 diabetes of >15 years' duration

- Presence of any additional risk factor for coronary artery disease
- Presence of microvascular disease (retinopathy or nephropathy, including microalbuminuria)
- Peripheral vascular disease
- Autonomic neuropathy

This recommendation has been developed in view of the higher prevalence of sudden death (Balkau *et al.*, 1999) and silent ischaemia (Janand-Delenne *et al.*, 1999) in people with type 2 diabetes.

Silent myocardial infarction (SMI) has a reported prevalence ranging from 10 to 20% in populations with diabetes, compared to 1–4% in the general population. Variations in reported prevalence probably occur due to differences in populations studied, screening techniques used and diagnostic criteria. Janand-Delenne *et al.* (1999) conducted a cross-sectional study to estimate the prevalence of SMI in a population with diabetes and to determine a high-risk population. The authors screened 203 asymptomatic people with type 1 and type 2 diabetes using either an exercise test (positive test ≥ 1 mm ST depression), thallium myocardial scintography, or both, and confirmed by coronary angiography. The total prevalence of angiographically confirmed SMI was 4.8% (2.3% in males, 7.4% in females) in people with type 1 diabetes and 12.1% (20.9% in males, 3.4% in females) in people with type 2 diabetes. Male gender and the presence of retinopathy, PAD and a family history of coronary artery disease were predictive factors for SMI in people with type 2 diabetes.

It is important to note that the recommendation of pre-participation exercise screening in people with diabetes is not routinely followed in the UK. If resources are available, this screening process can provide valuable information. The exercise test should be performed to evaluate for ischaemia, arrhythmia, abnormal hypertensive response to exercise or abnormal orthostatic responses during or after exercise. The stress test also provides information regarding initial aerobic capacity, specific precautions that may need to be taken and heart rate or perceived exertion that could be used to prescribe activities.

Monitoring

Risks associated with physical activity for people with type 2 diabetes are sports-related injuries and hypoglycaemia. It has been suggested that people with diabetes engaging in physical activity, exercise and sport are more prone to musculoskeletal injuries than people without diabetes. This increased risk may be due to the presence of neuropathy, obesity and/or vascular disease. It is important that appropriate steps are taken to avoid injury during physical activity participation. These include setting realistic physical activity goals, with consideration given to appropriate intensity and duration, inclusion of an exercise warm-up and cool-down and stretching periods and encouragement of appropriate footwear.

The risk of hypoglycaemia applies to patients with type 2 diabetes who are treated with sulphonylureas or insulin, and is generally not an issue for those managed through diet and physical activity or metformin. Hypoglycaemia can occur during or soon after physical activity, or it may be delayed for up to 24 hours following a single session of strenuous exercise. The best way to avoid hypoglycaemia in those at risk is to encourage them to monitor blood glucose levels before, during (if the activity is of long duration) and after exercise. Advice can be given on supplementary consumption of food before and/or after exercise, and, if appropriate, the reduction of insulin dose prior to exercise. Specific advice can be obtained through consultation with the local diabetes centres.

The AACPR (2004) advised that:

• the blood glucose level of the patient with diabetes must be under control before beginning an exercise programme;

• patients should not exercise if blood glucose levels are >300 mg/dL;

• an insulin-dependent patient should have a carbohydrate snack of 20–30 g before exercise if blood glucose is <100 mg/dL;

• blood glucose should be measured before, during and after exercise;

• adjustments in carbohydrate dose and/or insulin may be necessary before or after exercise.

It is most important that patients and staff are knowledgeable about the signs and symptoms of a hypoglycaemic attack. Prompt action in response to signs of weakness, faintness, sweating, pallor, confusion or belligerence can avoid a loss of consciousness. (See Thow, 2006, Ch. 6, pp. 174–5, for more on care of patients with diabetes.)

Improving exercise adherence for people with diabetes

Despite substantial evidence showing potential health benefits of frequent physical activity for people with type 2 diabetes, physical activity is rarely included as part of diabetes management. A survey of diabetes health care professionals showed that they spend little time educating patients about physical activity, and advice given is inadequate and unstructured (Berlanga *et al.*, 2000). The question of how to promote physical activity in people with type 2 diabetes has received little attention. The majority of research examining the effects of physical activity on diabetes management has used structured exercise programmes in which one exercise mode applies to all participants. Patient compliance in these studies is often disappointing, and no assessment of the effectiveness of these interventions in the long term has been made.

The position statement on exercise and type 2 diabetes published by the ACSM (2000) provides some information on ways to promote adoption and maintenance of physical activity in people with type 2 diabetes. The position statement highlights the use of the transtheoretical model of behaviour change (Prochaska and DiClemente, 1983) as a framework

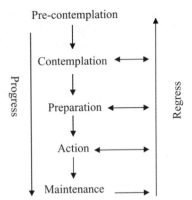

Figure 2.1 Stage of exercise behaviour change. (Adapted from Proshaska and DiClemente, 1983, and Marcus *et al.*, 1992.)

for describing and predicting behaviour change. This model, illustrated in Figure 2.1, was adapted to exercise by Marcus and colleagues in 1992, and has encouraged in recent years the use of physical activity interventions tailored to the specific needs of the individual.

The stage of change model proposes that individuals move through five stages of change when adopting a new behaviour. These stages have been labelled as follows: pre-contemplation (do not intend to change), contemplation (intend to change), preparation (have made some changes), action (actively engaging in a new behaviour) and maintenance (sustaining change over time). Progression from one stage to another is not always linear, and at any point individuals can relapse to a previous stage. The stage of change model can be used to assess an individual's motivational readiness to become more active and as a means of selecting appropriate cognitive behaviour strategies for the promotion of physical activity. Table 2.3 describes appropriate strategies to promote physical activity during each stage of exercise behaviour change. (See Thow, 2006, Ch. 8, for more information on maintaining physical activity.)

Table 2.3 Appropriate strategies during each stage of exercise behaviour change.

Stage of exercise behaviour change	Appropriate strategy
Pre-contemplation	Increase awareness of benefits of activity and risks of inactivity in people with diabetes
Contemplation	Evaluation of expected or experienced benefits and costs of behaviour change for people with diabetes
Preparation	Finding appropriate activities, realistic goal setting and developing social support for people with diabetes
Action	Rewarding achievements, overcoming barriers for people with diabetes
Maintenance	Varying activities, planning ahead to stay active for people with diabetes

Physical activity consultation is a relatively new cognitive behaviour intervention developed by Loughlan and Mutrie (1995, 1997). Similar to motivational interviewing, physical activity consultation is an individualised counselling intervention that incorporates reflective listening, reviewing current physical activity behaviour, decisional balancing, social support and the development of realistic physical activity goals.

There are several important differences between the two interventions. Motivational interviewing is aimed primarily at individuals in pre-contemplation or contemplation stages of behaviour change. Miller and Rollnick (2001) state that motivational interviewing is most effective to 'start the process of change' and that additional strategies are required to 'make the change'. Physical activity consultation, in comparison, is aimed at individuals in contemplation and preparation stages of behaviour change, in other words, individuals who are ready to change exercise behaviour. During physical activity consultation the counsellor gives advice to the client, whereas during motivational interviewing the counsellor plays a passive role and encourages the participant to present his or her own arguments and strategies for change.

Physical activity consultation for people with diabetes

Current research provides modest support for the use of physical activity consultation for physical activity promotion in populations with diabetes. Two randomised controlled pilot studies demonstrated physical activity consultation to be effective for promoting short-term (1 month) physical activity in people with type 1 (Hasler et al., 2000) and type 2 diabetes (Kirk et al., 2001). Kirk et al. (2003, 2004) identified the effectiveness of physical activity consultation for promotion of physical activity in people with type 2 diabetes over periods of 6 and 12 months. Participants assigned to the intervention group received a physical activity consultation at baseline and 6 months, with supporting phone calls 1 and 3 months after each consultation. Participants in the control group received the standard, usual care, exercise and diabetes leaflet. Outcome measures taken at baseline, at 6 months and at 12 months included parameters of physical activity (self-report questionnaire, activity monitor, stage and processes of exercise behaviour change), physiological variables (blood pressure, body mass index, cardiorespiratory fitness), biochemical variables (HbA_{1c}, full lipid profile, fibrinogen) and parameters of quality of life. In comparison to the control group, participants receiving the physical activity consultation intervention demonstrated consistent improvements in both subjective and objective measures of physical activity levels, progression in stage of exercise behaviour change, and an increase in the frequency of using the ten processes of behaviour change. From baseline to 6 and 12 months an average increase of 150 and 130 minutes, respectively, of moderate-to-vigorous physical activity was recorded by the intervention group. Favourable effects were also recorded in glycaemic control, cardiorespiratory fitness, blood pressure, total cholesterol and a small number of quality-of-life parameters. Throughout the study period, the control group recorded a decrease in physical activity levels and deterioration in glycaemic control. This finding highlights the argument that basic educational exercise and diabetes leaflets, often used in current routine care, are not effective in stimulating physical activity behaviour change in people with type 2 diabetes. This suggests that awareness of desired health practices is not sufficient for bringing about the adoption of health behaviour change.

In a similar study, Chun-Ja *et al.* (2004) investigated the effectiveness of physical activity consultation, based on the transtheoretical model of behaviour change and tailored to stage of change, over a 3-month period. This study used a control group who received the usual educational advice. Again, the intervention group, compared to the control group, showed significant improvements in stage of exercise behaviour change, physical activity levels, fasting blood glucose and HbA_{1c}. The control group in this study recorded no significant changes. Di Loreto *et al.* (2003) demonstrated effective physical activity promotion over 2 years in people with type 2 diabetes using brief physician-based physical activity counselling. The intervention used in this study was individualised and incorporated cognitive behavioural strategies, similar to those previously described. In contrast, the intervention was not tailored to stage of exercise behaviour change. Each intervention participant received a physical activity consultation at baseline, and this was supported with a phone call 1 month later and with appointments at the diabetes outpatient clinic every 3 months. The control group received usual care in the form of general educational advice. After 2 years the intervention group recorded a sevenfold increase in physical activity levels, in addition to a significant decrease in body mass index and HbA_{1c}. The control group recorded a significant increase in body mass index and no significant changes in physical activity levels or $HbA_{1c.}$ A post hoc analysis of the intervention demonstrated that the greater the amount of energy expenditure due to leisure time physical activity, the greater the beneficial effects on several biological parameters and cost savings.

A randomised pilot study examined the effectiveness of adding motivational interviewing strategies to a behavioural weight control programme for women with type 2 diabetes (Smith *et al.*, 1997). Participants who received motivational interviewing strategies had significantly better attendance, submitted more self-monitoring diaries, monitored their blood glucose more often and achieved better glucose control following treatment. Self-reported frequency of exercise and recording of caloric intake also improved, although not significantly.

Providing physical activity consultation for patients with diabetes within CR provides a way of individualising the prescription and education of patients, and may help to increase the adherence of people with diabetes to these programmes. In the general population, physical activity consultation has been delivered through a range of formats including face-to-face contact, group sessions and medicated channels such as telephone or the internet. In diabetes populations, the majority of physical activity consultation interventions have been delivered through face-to-face contact. This method of delivery can be time-consuming and there is often confusion over who is the best person to deliver these interventions. Future research should investigate the effectiveness of other methods of delivery of physical activity consultation in diabetes populations.

Key messages

• There will be more overweight/obese and type 2 diabetic participants in CR in the near future.
• People with type 2 diabetes and CR exercise professionals must be diligent in monitoring blood sugar levels and have emergency procedures in place for hypoglycaemia.
• There must be vigilance on foot care and immediate action on any sign of deterioration.
• Habitual exercise has considerable physiological and psychological benefits to the people with diabetes.
• Exercise behaviour change interventions should focus on enhancing the self-efficacy of people with diabetes/overweight subjects.
• People with type 2 diabetes should aim for a caloric expenditure of 1000 kcal/week and for weight loss of ≤2000 kcal/week.
• Exercise professionals must provide alternative exercise prescription for complications of diabetes.

Summary and conclusions

A substantial amount of evidence supports the theory that regular, frequent exercise has the potential to provide important health benefits for people with type 2 diabetes. What remains unclear is how physical activity can be promoted in this population over the long term. In view of the complexity of type 2 diabetes, its complications and their effect on exercise capacity, an individualised physical activity prescription is undoubtedly required. Individualised physical activity prescription, taking into account existing medical complications, will maximise the benefits of physical activity and minimise the risks. This in turn will enhance adherence.

It is crucial that physical activity behaviour changes are maintained, as people with diabetes appear to have more barriers to activity. Although structured exercise programmes have been shown to be effective in the short term at increasing physical activity levels and providing important health benefits, these programmes are often time-consuming, reach a limited number of people and are relatively ineffective in the long term.

Interventions that help people with type 2 diabetes to become more physically active and maintain this behaviour change in the long term are required.

Cognitive behavioural interventions, such as motivational interviewing and physical activity consultation, have increasingly been shown to be effective at promoting and maintaining physical activity behaviour in the general population. These interventions have potential to be effective in a diabetes population. These interventions allow for an individualised exercise prescription, taking into account the individual's disease and motivational state. Cognitive behavioural strategies can be developed to maintain physical activity behaviour change, and education can be given to avoid any complications of exercise in diabetes.

Finally, these interventions are relatively inexpensive and could reach a large number of people. With minimal training, these behaviour change interventions could be conducted by any one of the CR or diabetes care team.

References

Albright, A. (1998) Exercise precautions and recommendations for patients with autonomic neuropathy. *Diabetes Spectrum*, 11, 231–7.

Aliev, T., Abdullaev, N., Mirza-Zade, V., *et al*. (1993) Role of exercise in rehabilitation of coronary heart disease in cases combined with non insulin-dependent diabetes mellitus. *Sports Medicine Training and Rehabilitation*, 4, 53–5.

American Association of Cardiovascular and Pulmonary Rehabilitation (AACPR) (2004) *Guidelines for Cardiac Rehabilitation and Secondary Prevention Programmes*, 4th edn. Champaign, IL: Human Kinetics.

American College of Sports Medicine (ACSM) (1990) Position stand on the recommended quality and quantity of exercise for developing and maintaining cardiorespiratory and muscular fitness in health adults. *Medicine and Science in Sports and Exercise*, 22, 265–74.

American College of Sports Medicine (ACSM) (2000) Exercise and type 2 diabetes. *Medicine and Science in Sports and Exercise*, 32, 1345–60.

American College of Sports Medicine (ACSM) (2006) *Guidelines for Exercise Testing and Prescription*, 7th edn. Baltimore, MD: Lippincott, Williams & Wilkins.

American Diabetes Association (ADA) (2001) Diabetes mellitus and exercise. *Diabetes Care*, 24, S51.

Amos, A.F., McCarty, D.J., Zimmet, P. (1997) The rising global burden of diabetes and its complications: estimates and projections to the year 2010. *Diabetic Medicine*, 14, S7–85.

Ary, D., Toobert, D., Wilson, W., *et al*. (1986) Patient perspective on factors contributing to nonadherence to diabetes regimens. *Diabetes Care*, 9, 168–72.

Balkau, B., Jouven, X., Ducimetiere, P., *et al*. (1999) Diabetes as a risk factors for sudden death. *Lancet*, 354, 1968–9.

Barnard, J., Jung, T., Inkeles, S. (1994) Diet and exercise in the treatment of NIDDM. *Diabetes Care*, 17, 1469–72.

Berlanga, F., Eltringham-Cox, A., Burr, W., *et al.* (2000) Physical activity in type 2 diabetes. Its role and the current care pattern: a survey of diabetes health care professionals in the UK. *Practical Diabetes International*, 17, 60–61.

Bernbaum, M., Albert, S., Cohen, J., *et al.* (1989) Cardiovascular conditioning in individuals with diabetic retinopathy. *Diabetes Care*, 12, 740–42.

Blair, S.N., Church, T.S. (2004) The fitness, obesity, and health equation: is physical activity the common denominator? *Journal of the American Medical Association*, 292(10), 1232–40.

Blair, S.N., Kampert, J., Kohl, H., *et al.* (1996) Influences of cardiorespiratory fitness and other precursors on cardiovascular disease and all-cause mortality in men and women. *Journal of the American Medical Association*, 276, 205–10.

Borg, G.A.V. (1982) Psychophysical bases of perceived exertion. *Medicine and Science in Sports and Exercise*, 14, 377–81.

Boulé, N.G., Haddad, E., Kenny G.P., *et al.* (2001) Effects of exercise on glycemic control and body mass in type 2 diabetes mellitus: a meta-analysis of controlled clinical trials. *Journal of the American Medical Association*, 286, 1218–27.

Brandenburg, S., Reush, J., Bauer, T., *et al.* (1999) Effect of exercise training on oxygen uptake kinetic responses in women with type 2 diabetes. *Diabetes Care*, 22, 1640–46.

Braun, B., Zimmermann, M., Kretchmer, N. (1995) Effects of exercise intensity on insulin sensitivity in women with non-insulin-dependent diabetes mellitus. *Journal of Applied Physiology*, 78, 300–306.

Calle-Pascual, A., Martin-Alvarez, P., Reyes, C., *et al.* (2001) Regular physical activity and reduced occurrence of microalbuminuria in type 2 diabetic patients. *Diabetes and Metabolism*, 19, 304–9.

Chun, B., Dobson, A., Heller, R. (1997) The impact of diabetes on survival among patients with first myocardial infarction. *Diabetes Care*, 20, 704–8.

Chun, D., Vaccarino, V., Murillo, J., *et al.* (2002) Cardiac outcomes after myocardial infarction in elderly patients with diabetes mellitus. *American Journal of Critical Care*, 11, 504–19.

Chun-Ja, K., Ae-Ran, H., Ji-Soo, Y. (2004) The impact of a stage matched intervention to promote exercise behaviour in participants with type 2 diabetes. *International Journal of Nursing Studies*, 41, 833–41.

Cruickshanks, K., Moss, S., Klein, R., *et al.* (1992) Physical activity and proliferative retinopathy in people diagnosed with diabetes before age 30 years. *Diabetes Care*, 15, 1267–72.

Dahlquist, G., Aperia, A., Carlsso, L., *et al.* (1983) Effect of metabolic control and duration on exercise induced albuminuria in diabetic teenagers. *Acta Paediatrica Scandinavia*, 72, 895–902.

Devlin, J., Hirshman, M., Horton, E., *et al.* (1987) Enhanced peripheral and splanchnic insulin sensitivity in NIDDM men after single bout of exercise. *Diabetes*, 36, 434–9.

Di Loreto, C.D., Fanelli, C., Lucidi, P., *et al.* (2003) Validation of a counselling strategy to promote the adoption and the maintenance of physical activity by type 2 diabetic subjects. *Diabetes Care*, 26, 404–8.

Diabetes UK (2007) *Reports and Statistics* (2004 edn). Available from http://www.diabetes.org.uk (accessed 5 December 2007).

Dishman, R.K., Ickes, W. (1981) Self-motivation and adherence to therapeutic exercise. *Journal of Behavioural Medicine*, 4, 421–38.

Donnan, P., Boyle, D., Broomhall, J., *et al*. (2002) Prognosis following first acute myocardial infarction in type 2 diabetes: a comparative population study. *Diabetic Medicine*, 19, 448–55.

Eriksson, J., Taimela, S., Eriksso, K., *et al*. (1997) Resistance training in the treatment of non-insulin dependent diabetes mellitus. *International Journal of Sports Medicine*, 18, 242–6.

Fisher, B.M., Shaw, K.M. (2001) Diabetes – state of premature cardiovascular death. *Practical Diabetes International*, 18, 183–4.

Ford, E., Herman, W. (1995) Leisure-time physical activity patterns in the U.S. diabetic population: findings from the 1990 National Health Interview Survey. *Diabetes Care*, 18, 27–33.

Franklin, B.A., Gordon, N.F. (2005) *Contemporary Diagnosis and Management in Cardiovascular Disease*. Newtown, PA: Handbooks in Health Care.

Fujinuma, H., Abe, R., Yamazaki, T., *et al*. (1999) Effect of exercise training on doses of oral agents and insulin. *Diabetes Care*, 22, 1754–5.

Glacca, A., Groenewoud, Y., Tsui, E., *et al*. (1998) Glucose production, utilization, and cycling in response to moderate exercise in obese subjects with type 2 diabetes and mild hyperglycaemia. *Diabetes*, 47, 1763–70.

Glasgow, R., Ruggiero, L., Eakin, E., *et al*. (1997) Quality of life and associated characteristics in a large national sample of adults with diabetes. *Diabetes Care*, 20, 562–7.

Graham, C., McCarthey, P. (1990) Exercise options for persons with diabetic complications. *The Diabetes Educator*, 16, 212–20.

Gregg, E.W., Gerzoff, R.B., Caspersen, C.J., *et al*. (2003). Relationship of walking to mortality among US adults with diabetes. *Archives of Internal Medicine*, 163, 1440–47.

Guion, W.K., Carter, C.A., Corwin, S.J. (2000) Knowledge of exercise in patients with diabetes mellitus. *Medicine and Science in Sports and Exercise*, 31, S361.

Gustafsson, I., Hildebrandt, P., Seibaek, M., *et al*. (2000) Long-term prognosis of diabetic patients with myocardial infarction: relation to antidiabetic treatment regimen. *European Heart Journal*, 21, 1937–43.

Haffner, S., Lehto, S., Ronnemaa, T., *et al*. (1998) Mortality from coronary heart disease in subjects with type 2 diabetes and in nondiabetic subjects with and without prior myocardial infarction. *New England Journal of Medicine*, 339, 229–34.

Hasler, T., Fisher, B., MacIntyre, P., *et al*. (2000) Exercise consultation and physical activity in patients with type 1 diabetes. *Practical Diabetes International*, 17, 44–8.

Hays, L., Clark, D. (1999) Correlates pf physical activity in a sample of older adults with type 2 diabetes. *Diabetes Care*, 22, 706–12.

Heath, G., Gavin, J., Hinderliter, J., *et al*. (1983) Effects of exercise and lack of exercise on glucose tolerance and insulin sensitivity. *Journal of Applied Physiology*, 55, 512–17.

Hiatt, W., Regensteiner, J., Hargarten, M., *et al*. (1989) Benefit of exercise conditioning for patients with peripheral arterial disease. *Circulation*, 81, 602–9.

Hilstead, J., Galbo, H., Christensen, N. (1979) Impaired cardiovascular responses to graded exercise in diabetic autonomic neuropathy. *Diabetes*, 28, 313–19.

Honkola, A., Forsen, T., Eriksson, J. (1997) Resistance training improves the metabolic profile in individuals with type 2 diabetes. *Acta Diabetologica*, 34, 245–8.

Ishii, T., Yamakita, T., Sato, T., *et al.* (1998) Resistance training improves insulin sensitivity in NIDDM subjects without altering maximal oxygen uptake. *Diabetes Care*, 21, 1353–5.

Janand-Delenne, B., Savin, B., Habib, G., *et al.* (1999) Silent myocardial ischemia in patients with diabetes. *Diabetes Care*, 22, 1396–400.

Kahn, J., Sisson, J., Vinik A. (1986) QT interval prolongation and sudden cardiac death in diabetic autonomic neuropathy. *Journal of Clinical Endocrinology and Metabolism*, 64, 751–4.

Kannel, W., McGee, D. (1979) Diabetes and glucose tolerance as risk factors for cardiovascular disease: the Framingham Study. *Diabetes Care*, 2, 20–26.

Karvonen, M.J., Kentala, F., Mustala O. (1957) The effects of training on heart rate: a longitudinal study. *Annales Medicinae Experimentalis et Biologiae Fenniae*, 35, 307–15.

Katoh, J., Hara, Y., Kurusu, M., *et al.* (1996) Cardiorespiratory function as assessed by exercise testing in patients with non-insulin-dependent diabetes mellitus. *The Journal of International Medical Research*, 24, 209–13.

Kevorkian, G. (1986) Effects of exercise on the insulin levels in diabetics. *Journal of Visual Impairment and Blindness*, 80, 954–5.

Khan, S., Rupp, J. (1995) The effect of exercise conditioning, diet, and drug therapy on glycosylated hemoglobin levels in type 2 (NIDDM) diabetics. *The Journal of Sports Medicine and Physical Fitness*, 35, 281–8.

King, A.C., Blair, S.N., Bild, D.E., *et al.* (1992) Determinants of physical activity and interventions in adults. *Medicine and Science in Sports and Exercise*, 24, S221–36.

Kingery, P., Glasgow, R. (1989) Self-efficacy and outcomes expectations in the self-regulation of non-insulin dependent diabetes mellitus. *Health Education*, 20, 13–19.

Kirk, A., Higgins, L., Hughes, A., *et al.* (2001) A randomised, controlled trial to study the effect of exercise consultation on the promotion of physical activity in people with type 2 diabetes: a pilot study. *Diabetic Medicine*, 18, 877–83

Kirk, A., Mutrie, N., MacIntyre, P., *et al.* (2003) Increasing physical activity in people with type 2 diabetes. *Diabetes Care*, 26, 1186–92.

Kirk, A., Mutrie, N., MacIntyre, P., *et al.* (2004) Effects of a 12-month physical activity consultation intervention on glycaemic control and on the status of cardiovascular risk factors in people with type 2 diabetes. *Diabetologica*, 47, 821–32.

Kjaer, M., Hollenbeck, C., Frey-Hewitt, B., *et al.* (1990) Glucoregulation and hormonal responses to maximal exercise in non-insulin-dependent diabetes. *Journal of Applied Physiology*, 68, 2067–74.

Knowler, W.C., Barrett-Connor, E., Fowler, S.E., *et al.* (2002) Diabetes prevention program research group. Reduction in the incidence of type 2 diabetes with lifestyle intervention or metformin. *New England Journal of Medicine*, 346, 393–403.

Kohl, H., Gordon, N., Villegas, J., *et al.* (1992) Cardiorespiratory fitness, glycemic status, and mortality risk in men. *Diabetes Care*, 15, 184–91.

Krug, L., Haire-Joshu, D., Heady, S. (1991) Exercise habits and exercise relapse in persons with non-insulin-dependent diabetes mellitus. *The Diabetes Educator*, 17, 185–8.

Larsen, J., Dela, F., Kjaer, M., *et al.* (1997) The effect of moderate exercise on postprandial glucose homeostasis in NIDDM patients. *Diabetologia*, 40, 447–53.

Lehmann, R., Vokac, A., Niedermann, K., *et al.* (1995) Loss of abdominal fat and improvement of the cardiovascular risk profile by regular moderate exercise training in patients with NIDDM. *Diabetologia*, 38, 1313–19.

Lehto, S., Pyorala, K., Miettinen, H., *et al.* (1994) Myocardial infarct size and mortality in patients with non-insulin-dependent diabetes mellitus. *Journal of Internal Medicine*, 236, 291–7.

Liang, P., Hughes, V., Fukagaw, V., *et al.* (1997) Increased prevalence of mitochondrial DNA deletions in skeletal muscle of older individuals with impaired glucose tolerance: possible marker of glycaemic stress. *Diabetes*, 46, 920–23.

Ligtenberg, P., Hoekstra, J., Bol, E., *et al.* (1997) Effects of physical training on metabolic control in elderly type 2 diabetes mellitus patients. *Clinical Science*, 93, 127–35.

Ligtenberg, P.C., Godaert, G.L.R., Hillenaar, F., *et al.* (1998) Influence of a physical training program on psychological well-being in elderly type 2 diabetes patients. *Diabetes Care*, 21, 2196–7.

Loughlan, C., Mutrie, N. (1995) Conducting an exercise consultation: guidelines for health professionals. *Journal of the Institute of Health Education*, 33, 78–82.

Loughlan, C., Mutrie, N. (1997) An evaluation of the effectiveness of the three interventions in promoting physical activity in a sedentary population. *Health Education Journal*, 65, 154–65.

Lowel, H., Koenig, W., Engel, S., *et al.* (2000) The impact of diabetes mellitus on survival after myocardial infarction: can it be modified by drug therapy? *Diabetologia*, 43, 218–26.

Lucas, B., Casillas, J., Verges, B., *et al.* (2000) Does diabetes affect results of cardiac rehabilitation? *Archives des Maladies du Coeur et des Vaisseaux*, 93, 263–9.

Mak, K., Moliterno, D., Granger, C., *et al.* (1997) Influence of diabetes mellitus on clinical outcomes in the thrombolytic era of acute myocardial infarction. *Journal of the American College of Cardiology*, 30, 171–9.

Malmberg, K., Yusuf, S., Gerstein, H., *et al.* (2000) Impact of diabetes on long term prognosis in patients with unstable angina and non Q wave myocardial infarction: results from the OASIS registry. *Circulation*, 102, 1014–19.

Marcus, B., Rossi, J., Selby, V., *et al.* (1992) The stages and processes of exercise adoption and maintenance in a worksite sample. *Health Psychology*, 11, 386–95.

Marsden, E. (1996) *The Role of Exercise in the Well-Being of People with Insulin Dependent Diabetes Mellitus: Perceptions of Patients and Health Professionals*, Thesis/Dissertation. Glasgow: University of Glasgow.

Martin, J.E., Dubbert, P.M., Katell, A.D., *et al.* (1984) Behavioural control of exercise in sedentary adults. *Journal of Consulting and Clinical Psychology*, 52, 795–811.

Melchior, T., Gadsboll, N., Hildebrandt, P., *et al.* (1996) Clinical characteristics, left and right ventricular ejection fraction, and long-term prognosis in patients with non-insulin dependent diabetes surviving an acute myocardial infarction. *Diabetic Medicine*, 13, 450–56.

Milani, R., Lavie, C. (1996) Behavioural differences and effects of cardiac rehabilitation in diabetic patients following cardiac events. *American Journal of Medicine*, 100, 517–23.

Miller, W., Rollnick, S. (2001) *Motivational Interviewing: Preparing People to Change Addictive Behavior*. New York: The Guilford Press.

Ming, W., Gibbons, L., Kampert, J., *et al.* (2000) Low cardiorespiratory fitness and physical inactivity as predictors of mortality in men with type 2 diabetes. *Annals of Internal Medicine*, 132, 605–11.

Minuk, H., Vranic, M., Marliss, E., *et al.* (1981) Glucoregulatory and metabolic response to exercise in obese non insulin diabetes. *American Journal of Physiology*, 240, E458–64.

Mogensen, C. (1995) Nephropathy: early. In: Ruderman, N., Devlin, J. (eds), *The Health Professionals Guide to Diabetes and Exercise*. Alexandria, VA: American Diabetes Association, pp. 164–74.

Moore, P. (2000) Type 2 diabetes is a major drain on resources. *British Medical Journal*, 320, 732.

Mourier, A., Gautier, J., Kerviler, E., *et al.* (1997) Mobilization of visceral adipose tissue related to the improvement in insulin sensitivity in response to physical training in NIDDM. *Diabetes Care*, 20, 385–91.

Mukamal, K., Nesto, R., Cohe, M., *et al.* (2001) Impact of diabetes on long-term survival after acute myocardial infarction: comparability of risk with prior myocardial infarction. *Diabetes Care*, 24, 1422–7.

Padgett, D. (1991) Correlates of self-efficacy beliefs among patients with non-insulin dependent diabetes mellitus in Zagreb, Yugoslavia. *Patient Education and Counselling*, 18, 139–47.

Pate, R., Pratt, M., Blair, S., *et al.* (1995) Physical activity and public health: a recommendation from the Centers for Disease Control and Prevention and the American College of Sports Medicine. *Journal of the American Medical Association*, 273, 402–7.

Prochaska, J., DiClemente, C. (1983) Stages and processes of self-change in smoking: towards an integrative model of change. *Journal of Consulting and Clinical Psychology*, 51, 390–95.

Raz, I., Hause, E., Bursztyn, M. (1994) Moderate exercise improves glucose metabolism in uncontrolled elderly patients with non-insulin-dependent diabetes mellitus. *Israel Journal of Medical Sciences*, 30, 766–70.

Regensteiner, J., Bauer, T., Reush, J., *et al.* (1998) Abnormal oxygen uptake kinetic response in women with type II diabetes mellitus. *Journal of Applied Physiology*, 85, 310–17.

Regensteiner, J., Sippel, J., McFarling, *et al.* (1994) Effects of non-insulin-dependent diabetes on oxygen consumption during treadmill exercise. *Medicine and Science in Sports and Exercise*, 27, 875–81.

Rosengren, A., Spetz, C., Koster, M., *et al.* (2001) Sex differences in survival after myocardial infarction in Sweden. *European Heart Journal*, 22, 314–22.

Rosenstock, I.M. (1974) Historical origins of the health belief model. *Health Education Monographs*, 2, 1–9.

Roy, T., Peterson, H., Snider, H., *et al.* (1989) Autonomic influence on cardiovascular performance in diabetic subjects. *The American Journal of Medicine*, 87, 382–8.

Scottish Intercollegiate Guidelines Network (2001) *SIGN Guideline No. 55: Management of Diabetes – A National Clinical Guideline*. Edinburgh: Scottish Intercollegiate Guidelines Network.

Scottish Intercollegiate Guidelines Network (2006) *SIGN Guideline 89: Diagnosis and Management of Peripheral Arterial Disease*. Edinburgh: Scottish Intercollegiate Guidelines Network.

Simoneau, J., Kelley, D. (1997) Altered glycolytic and oxidative capacities of skeletal muscle contribute to insulin resistance in NIDDM. *Journal of Applied Physiology*, 83, 166–71.

Skarfors, E., Wegener, T., Selinus, I. (1987) Physical training as treatment for type 2 (non-insulin-dependent) diabetes in elderly men. A feasibility study over 2 years. *Diabetologia*, 30, 930–33.

Smith, D., Heckemeyer, C., Kratt, P., *et al.* (1997) Motivational interviewing to improve adherence to a behavioural weight-control program for older obese women with NIDDM. *Diabetes Care*, 20, 52–4.

Stewart, A., Hays, R., Wells, K., *et al.* (1994) Long-term functioning and well-being outcomes associated with physical activity and exercise in patients with chronic conditions in the medical outcomes study. *Journal of Clinical Epidemiology*, 47, 719–30.

Suresh, V., Harrison, R., Houghton, P., *et al.* (2001) Standard cardiac rehabilitation is less effective for diabetics. *International Journal of Clinical Practice*, 55, 445–8.

Swift, C., Armstrong, J., Beerman, K., *et al.* (1995) Attitudes and beliefs about exercise among persons with non-insulin-dependent diabetes. *The Diabetes Educator*, 21, 533–40.

Taniguchi, A., Fukushima, M., Sakai, M., *et al.* (2000) Effect of physical training on insulin sensitivity in Japanese type 2 diabetic patients. *Diabetes Care*, 23, 857–60.

Tantucci, C., Bottini, P., Dottorini, L., *et al.* (1996) Ventilatory response to exercise in diabetic subjects with autonomic neuropathy. *Journal of Applied Physiology*, 81, 1978–86.

Thompson, P.D., Crouse, S.F., Goodaste, B.R., *et al.* (2001) The acute versus chronic responses to exercise. *Medicine and Science in Sports and Exercise*, 33(60), 438–45.

Thow, M. (2006) *Exercise Leadership in Cardiac Rehabilitation an Evidence Based Approach*. Chichester, England: Wiley.

Trovati, M., Carta, Q., Cavalot, F., *et al.* (1984) Influence of physical training on blood glucose control, glucose tolerance, insulin secretion, and insulin action in non-insulin dependent diabetic patients. *Diabetes Care*, 7, 416–20.

Tuomilehto, J., Lindstrom, J., Eriksson, J., *et al.* (2001) Prevention of type 2 diabetes mellitus by changes in lifestyle among subjects with impaired glucose tolerance. *New England Journal of Medicine*, 344, 1343–50.

United Kingdom Prospective Diabetes Study Group (UKPDSG) (2002) Tight blood pressure control and the risk of macrovascular and microvascular complications in type 2 diabetes UKPDS 38. *British Medical Journal*, 317, 703–13.

Usui, K., Yamanouchi, K., Asai, K., *et al.* (1998) The effect of low intensity bicycle exercise on the insulin-induced glucose uptake in obese patients with type 2 diabetes. *Diabetes Research and Clinical Practice*, 41, 57–61.

Vanninen, E., Uusitupa, M., Remes, J., *et al.* (1992) Relationship between hyperglycaemia and aerobic power in men with newly diagnosed type 2 (non insulin-dependent) diabetes. *Clinical Physiology*, 12, 667–77.

Verges, B., Patois-Verges, B., Lucas, B., *et al.* (2001) Effect of cardiac rehabilitation after an ischaemic heart event on cardiovascular capacities, in type 2 diabetes. *Diabetologia*, 44, 261.

Walker, K., Piers, L., Putt, R., *et al.* (1999) Effects of regular walking on cardiovascular risk factors and body composition in normoglycemic women and women with type 2 diabetes. *Diabetes Care*, 22, 555–61.

Wallace, J. (ed.) (1997) Obesity. In: American College of Sports Medicine. *Exercise Management for Persons with Chronic Diseases and Disabilities*. Leeds: Human Kinetics, pp. 106–11.

Wankel, L.M. (1984) Decision-making and social-support strategies for increasing exercise involvement. *Journal of Cardiac Rehabilitation*, 4, 124–35.

Wei, M., Gibbons, L., Mitchell, T., *et al.* (1999) The association between cardiorespiratory fitness and impaired fasting glucose and type 2 diabetes mellitus in men. *Annals of Internal Medicine*, 130, 89–96.

Weyer, C., Linkeschowa, R., Heise, T., *et al.* (1998) Implications of the traditional and the new ACSM physical activity recommendations on weight reduction in dietary treated obese subjects. *International Journal of Obesity*, 22, 1071–8.

Wilson, W., Ary, D., Bigard, A., *et al.* (1986) Psychosocial predictors of self-care behaviours (compliance) and glycemic control in non-insulin-dependent diabetes mellitus. *Diabetes Care*, 9, 614–22.

World Health Organization (WHO) (1999) Definition, diagnosis and classification of diabetes mellitus and its complications. Report of a WHO consultation. Geneva, Switzerland: Department of Non-communicable Disease Surveillance.

3 | Chronic Heart Failure

Ann Taylor and Aynsley Cowie

Chapter outline

Over the past years we have seen an increasing number of people with chronic (or congestive) heart failure (CHF). This increase is primarily due to the increase in the age of the population and in survivors of myocardial infarction. There is compelling evidence that people with this condition can benefit physiologically and psychosocially from participation in regular exercise. It is therefore important for health professionals working in cardiac rehabilitation to be aware of the current literature and guidelines surrounding exercise and CHF. This chapter outlines the pathophysiology of CHF, describes its management through physical activity and exercise, and provides guidelines on exercise prescription for this population.

Features of chronic heart failure

People with CHF commonly experience decreased exercise tolerance and increased shortness of breath, and regular exercise has a role in reducing the effect of these factors and improving quality of life. The levels of functional activity in this group form the basis of the New York Heart Association (NYHA) classification of symptoms (Remme and Swedberg, 2001), which is widely used in clinical practice and research literature (see Box 3.1). The clinical features associated with CHF arise from impaired blood flow due to an inadequate myocardial function, which is unable to meet the metabolic demands of the body, together with concomitant widespread multisystemic involvement (Chong and Lip, 2007).

Distinctions have been made between systolic and diastolic cardiac impairment within CHF. Systolic heart failure is characterised by reduced left ventricular ejection fraction (LVEF), increased end-diastolic volume and normal/reduced stroke volume. However, over half of the patient population have a normal LVEF and are described as having diastolic heart failure (Quinones *et al.*, 2006). The mechanism of the latter is poorly understood, and may be related to an active fibrotic process which increases ventricular stiffness, leading to compromised filling (Martos, 2007). For more on diastolic heart failure and its mechanisms, Zile and LeWinter (2007) provide an overview of the current issues associated with diastolic

Box 3.1 New York Heart Association classification of heart failure symptoms (Remme and Swedberg, 2001).

Class I	No limitations; ordinary physical activity does not cause undue fatigue, breathlessness or palpitations
Class II	Slight limitation of physical activity; comfortable at rest, ordinary physical activity (e.g. getting dressed) results in fatigue, breathlessness or palpitations
Class III	Marked limitation of physical activity; comfortable at rest, less than ordinary physical activity (e.g. walking on a flat surface) will lead to symptoms
Class IV	Inability to carry on any physical activity without discomfort; symptoms are present even at rest; with any physical activity, increased discomfort is experienced

malfunction. Although there is a difference in mortality between the two forms of CHF, with a mortality rate of 5–8% for diastolic heart failure and 10–15% for systolic heart failure (De Keulenaer and Brutsaert, 2007), the American College of Sports Medicine (ACSM, 2006) considers the effects to pathophysiology to be similar for both types.

Pathophysiology and incidence of CHF

Pathophysiology
Whilst reduced cardiac function is a feature of CHF, there is a poor relationship between left ventricular dysfunction and exercise tolerance (Cohn *et al.*, 1993). This highlights the complexity of the changes in physiology, which is a feature of CHF. Of particular interest to exercise professionals and those facilitating cardiac rehabilitation are changes within the vascular, respiratory and neurohumeral systems and changes in muscle function and structure, as these influence exercise performance. The changes may follow an ischaemic episode, that is, myocardial infarction, or have a non-ischaemic cardiac origin. The latter includes changes in the structure of cardiac valves, which may lead to restricted filling (mitral and tricuspid stenosis), pressure overload (aortic stenosis and hypertension) and volume loading due to valve incompetence.

There is also a strong relationship between the development of CHF and the presence of diabetes mellitus (Nichols, 2001). The Framingham Heart Study indicates that 12% of women and 6% of men have CHF, which is accounted for independently by diabetes mellitus, and it is considered a higher risk factor for ischaemic than non-ischaemic heart failure (Das, 2004). This may be due to the similarity of risk factors for the two disease states.

Systemic inflammation is also associated with heart failure, as indicated by increased levels of biochemical markers within the circulatory system (Chong and Lip, 2007). These include elevated levels of tissue factor (TF), vascular endothelial growth factor (VEGF), tumour necrosis factor alpha (TNFα) and interleukin (IL-1). This increase in prothrombic state is linked to the decreased myocardial contraction of heart failure and an imbalance between natural pro- and anticoagulants. The level of circulating endothelial cells is also raised when endothelial integrity becomes compromised. A worsening outcome in heart failure is associated with increased levels of C-reactive protein, which may increase the level of TNFα.

Changes in the cardiovascular system in CHF

People with CHF experience increased activity of the sympathetic nervous system as a compensatory mechanism to maintain cardiac output and blood pressure (Jackson et al., 2000). As the clinical state progresses this increase in activity becomes a dominant pathophysiological feature of CHF (Chwan et al., 2007; Piepoli and Coats, 1996), and together with changes in activity of the humeral system, it has widespread effects on the cardiovascular system, as outlined in Figure 3.1.

Overall, the presentation is of excessive sympathetic activity, resulting in increased heart rate and incidence of potentially fatal arrhythmias, vasoconstriction, increased end-diastolic volume and finally afterload increased demands on myocardial function, which is already compromised. Due to excessive sympathetic activity the baroreceptors become downregulated and uncoupled from their normal reflex and heart rate variability is reduced. The latter is often used as a marker for the activity of the autonomic nervous system in CHF, with a direct relationship existing between heart rate variability and improvement in clinical state (Nolan et al., 1998). The altered neurohumeral activity causes an overall increase in circulatory volume and resultant peripheral (and later pulmonary) oedema.

Changes in skeletal muscle in CHF

Numerous studies indicate that both the structure and the metabolism of skeletal muscle are altered in people with CHF, and this contributes to their reduced exercise tolerance (Harrington et al., 1997; Mancini et al., 1992; Schaulfelberger et al., 1997; van der Ent et al., 1998). The early onset of muscle fatigue associated with CHF is a result of changes in the profile of muscle fibres, whereby they are reduced in size, number and metabolic characteristics (Mettauer et al., 2006). There is a shift within muscles towards a predominance of the number of fibres that utilise anaerobic metabolism, and they show concomitant structural and metabolic changes that reflect this change in activity (Drexler et al., 1992; Poole-Wilson et al., 1992). These modifications are considered to be beyond that attributable to disuse atrophy (which may occur in the later stages of CHF) and have been found in both peripheral and respiratory muscles. Muscle apoptosis

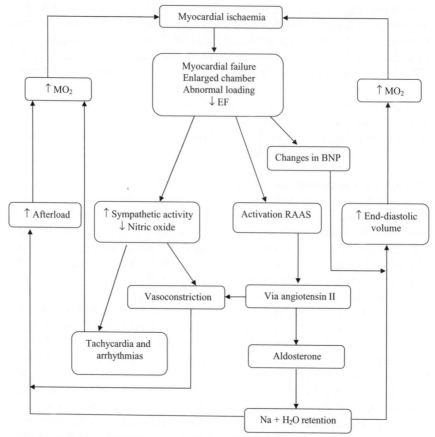

Figure 3.1 Outline of changes in the cardiovascular system. MO_2, myocardial oxygen demand; BNP, brain natriuretic peptide; RAAS, renin-angiotensin-aldosterone system; Na, sodium; H_2O, water; EF, ejection fraction. (↑↓ indicates increase or decrease.)

may be triggered by TNFα (Vescovo and Dalla Libera, 2006), and higher ergoreflex activity has been found to correlate with decreased muscle mass (Piepoli *et al.*, 2006).

Changes in respiratory system with CHF

Increased breathlessness is the other main factor that limits exercise tolerance. The inspiratory muscles show similar decreases in strength and endurance to that of peripheral muscles (Stassijns, 1996), and increased minute ventilation is primarily attributed to an increase in rate rather than depth of respiration (Dall'Ago *et al.*, 2006; Olson *et al.*, 2006). A disproportionate increase in minute ventilation in response to carbon dioxide production is considered to be a contributory factor to breathlessness (Guazzi *et al.*, 2007). This increase in demand on the musculature of the respiratory system, which has restricted scope to respond, adds to the work of breathing. There is some evidence that functional residual capacity is decreased in CHF as a result of pulmonary congestion, causing a mild restrictive respiratory pattern (Torchio *et al.*, 2006), and there is also a high incidence of sleep-disordered breathing (Oldenburg *et al.*, 2007). These respiratory features may be compounded by the presence of chronic airway obstruction, as the latter has been identified as the highest worldwide comorbidity factor for CHF (Lang and Mancini, 2007).

Pathophysiological changes in the cardiovascular, muscular and respiratory systems collectively contribute to the characteristic decrease in exercise tolerance, due to early onset of muscle fatigue, anaemia and high levels of breathlessness.

Incidence of CHF

There is an increasing prevalence of CHF with an ageing population and improved peri-infarction survival, with a resultant increase in the number of people with impaired ventricular function. This is reflected in changes in hospital admissions between 1990 and 2004 within the US, where hospitalisation for people following a myocardial infarction decreased by 8% but for those with CHF increased by 33%. During this period deaths from CHF rose by 28%. The Framingham Heart Study indicates a lifetime risk of 20% for developing CHF, and the incidence increases with age (Lloyd-Jones *et al.*, 2002). CHF is associated with a mortality rate of 1.7 years for men and 3.2 years for women from time of diagnosis (Lloyd-Jones *et al.*, 2002), with the highest rate occurring in NYHA class IV (Cohn *et al.*, 1993) and the lowest in people who remain ambulant (Carson *et al.*, 1996).

Many studies have investigated factors that may predict the progression of CHF, with the objective of directing management strategies to those prolonging life. Factors that have been suggested as predictors of a poor clinical outcome include low levels of activity (Ingle *et al.*, 2007, Passantino *et al.*, 2006), coexistence of diabetes mellitus (Kamalesh, 2006), shortness of breath at night (Javaheri *et al.*, 2007; Wang *et al.*, 2007), increased brain natriuretic peptide (Gademan *et al.*, 2007), decreased level of haemoglobin (Falk *et al.*, 2006; Mitchell, 2007), a body mass index below 22 kg/m^2 (Cicoira *et al.*, 2007; Goldberg *et al.*, 2007) and the presence of poor renal function (Lang and Mancini, 2007). However, as the variety of outcome predictors demonstrate, there is a lack of consensus regarding potential prognostic indicators, which may be a reflection on the multifactorial nature of the syndrome.

Benefits of exercise for CHF

Until the late twentieth century prolonged bed rest and avoidance of exercise was commonly recommended for people with CHF, thereby further decreasing their level of exercise tolerance. However, with an increasing body of evidence illustrating the potential benefits of regular exercise, clinical guidelines recommend that this group of people be encouraged to participate in exercise programmes (European Society of Cardiology (ESC), 2005; Hunt *et al.*, 2005 – American College of Cardiology/Heart Association; National Institute of Clinical Excellence, 2003; Scottish Intercollegiate Guidelines Network (SIGN), 2002). A challenge for those involved in delivering exercise programmes is the divergence of the clinical status of participants and the organisation of programmes cited in the research literature. Readers should consult the clinical guidelines for details of the format of exercise programmes on which their recommendations are based.

Of particular interest to the participant is the benefit of exercise on their functional activity, and a small improvement in exercise performance as a result of exercise training may have a major impact on their quality of life (Mathew, 1998). The physiological response to regular exercise for this patient group is similar to that for healthy people, but benefits are quickly lost on cessation of exercise (Coats *et al.*, 1992; Taylor, 1999). Improvements have been measured in aerobic function and muscle strength (You Fang, 2003), decrease in resting heart rate and heart rate recovery (Myers *et al.*, 2007), and improved endothelial function (Hambrecht *et al.*, 2000). These all contribute to an increase in activity, which may result in an improvement of NYHA class (Rees *et al.*, 2004) and also be predictive of improved prognosis. This improvement in activity is partially due to the influence of exercise on neurohumeral function, resulting in a decrease of abnormal sympathetic activity and improved cardiovascular function (Adamopoulos *et al.*, 2002; Conraads, 2002; Gademan *et al.*, 2007). Improvement in the latter allows muscle fibre type to assume a more normal metabolic profile and become less prone to early fatigue.

The effect of exercise training on cardiac function is equivocal. Where benefits have been identified they are considered to be secondary to improvements in vascular function (Hambrecht *et al.*, 2000). Improvements in myocardial perfusion and the reversal of remodelling have been measured following aerobic exercise (Belardinelli *et al.*, 1999; Haykowsky *et al.*, 2007). The relationship between minute ventilation and carbon dioxide production approaches more normal levels after a short period of exercise training (Coats *et al.*, 1992; Taylor, 1999), and specific respiratory muscle training results in changes in muscle function similar to other muscles (Johnson *et al.*, 1998; Weiner *et al.*, 1999). The effects of these changes on breathlessness are thought to be mainly derived through reduced sensitivity of receptors (Weiner *et al.*, 1999). There is some evidence to suggest that cardiac events are decreased following exercise training, but further studies are required to determine whether there is a beneficial effect on mortality (Belardinelli *et al.*, 1999; De Sutter *et al.*, 2005; Smart and Marwick, 2004; Whellan *et al.*, 2007).

Selection for exercise training with CHF

Although people with CHF have greater overall morbidity and mortality than those with most other forms of coronary heart disease (Konstantinos and Tokmakidis, 2005), they can participate in exercise rehabilitation, provided there is a well-defined, locally agreed recruitment and referral protocol (Department of Health, 2000). This protocol should incorporate clear inclusion and exclusion criteria and a thorough pre-exercise assessment (Association of Chartered Physiotherapists in Cardiac Rehabilitation, 2006).

Most evidence for exercise rehabilitation in CHF focuses on those symptomatically classified as NYHA class II or III (see Box 3.1). Clinical guidelines produced by the Working Group on Heart Failure of the ESC (2001) indicate that carefully selected individuals of NYHA class IV may participate in an appropriately prescribed exercise training programme, provided they are closely monitored throughout. Importantly, any dyspnoea at rest must be minimised with pharmacological therapy before training begins (Meyer *et al.*, 2004). No studies have been published evaluating the effects of training on people with unstable CHF (experiencing periods of cardiac decompensation), and it is advocated that people are clinically stable for 1 month prior to training (Mears, 2006). People with NYHA class IV CHF have rarely been included in research studies, but may derive physical and psychosocial benefit from training, and consequently should not be excluded from exercise programmes (Meyer *et al.*, 2004).

Recommendations for exercise training are generally aimed at people with an LVEF of below 40%. However, no minimal LVEF criterion for undertaking exercise has been agreed, and people with the lowest ejection fraction values may derive the greatest benefit from training. As there is little correlation between central cardiac function and exercise tolerance, an LVEF greater than 40% should not necessarily exclude someone from an exercise programme (ESC, 2001). Training gains do not appear to be dependent on the aetiology of CHF, and as with other cardiac populations, there has been little research to assess the benefit of exercise in elderly individuals and women (Rees *et al.*, 2004). Contraindications to exercise training are provided in Table 3.1 (ESC, 2001).

Assessment and risk stratification for CHF

It is widely accepted that impairment of left ventricular function is a strong predictor of a poorer prognosis in people with cardiac disease (Specchia *et al.*, 1996). According to criteria outlined by the American Association of Cardiovascular and Pulmonary Rehabilitation (AACVPR, 2006), people with LVEF below 40% are amongst those at higher risk of further cardiac events. During exercise, compromised cardiac output and ischaemic loading resulting from left ventricular dysfunction could potentially lead to a life-threatening arrhythmia (Belardinelli, 2003). Thorough pre-training

Table 3.1 Contraindications to exercise training for people with chronic heart failure.

Relative contraindications	Absolute contraindications
1.8 kg or more increase in body mass over previous 1–3 days	Progressive worsening of exercise tolerance or dyspnoea at rest or on exertion over previous 3–5 days
Concurrent continuous or intermittent dobutamine therapy	Significant ischaemia at low rates ($<$2 METs = $\sim$50 W)
	Uncontrolled diabetes
Decrease in systolic blood pressure with exercise	Acute systemic illness or fever
NYHA functional class IV	Recent embolism
Complex ventricular arrhythmias at rest or appearing with exertion	Thrombophlebitis
	Active pericarditis or myocarditis
Supine resting heart rate $\geq$100 beats/min	Moderate-to-severe aortic stenosis
	Regurgitant valvular heart disease requiring surgery
Pre-existing comorbidities	Myocardial infarction within previous 3 weeks
	New onset of atrial fibrillation

ESC (2001).

assessment will ascertain the relative extent of this risk and enable appropriate and safe exercise prescription.

Subjective and objective pre-training assessment should provide written evidence of cardiac symptoms, current medications, results of relevant investigations, past medical history and comorbidities, cardiovascular risk profile (including current physical activity level) and response to exercise (Association of Chartered Physiotherapists in Cardiac Rehabilitation (ACPICR), 2006; Smart *et al.*, 2003). Repeat assessment throughout, and on completion of, the training programme will facilitate patient safety and allow an evaluation of physiological and psychosocial outcomes from the exercise programme (ESC, 2001).

Symptoms of CHF or other cardiac states should be ascertained in order to allow differentiation from any new or worsening features that arise during the training programme or an exercise session. Whilst Smart *et al.* (2003) recommend that people are on optimal medication doses prior to commencing training, this may take several weeks or months and could considerably delay entry into a rehabilitation programme. A list of baseline medications (inclusive of current dosages and plans for uptitration) will enable anticipation of signs and symptoms that may develop as medication doses are increased (see section 'Medication Issues for CHF'). To complete baseline data, results of a recent echocardiograph or electrocardiograph should be obtained (ESC, 2001). The electrocardiograph will probably have abnormal features, and any arrhythmias should be thoroughly evaluated, and optimally controlled, before training commences. As shown in Table 3.1, training is not recommended in people with serious ventricular arrhythmias. Results of any planned investigations to assess the extent of coronary heart disease (e.g. coronary angiography) will provide information regarding further cardiovascular risk and be completed before training commences.

Baseline body weight, resting blood pressure and heart rate should be obtained at the pre-training assessment and the importance of daily monitoring of 'dry' weight (i.e. on waking, after urination and before consumption of any fluid) should be highlighted. Weight gain may indicate decompensation of stable CHF, which necessitates abstinence from training until fully compensated (see Table 3.1). The ESC (2001) advocates a pre-training blood test and full cardiology review. However, provided the assessment covers the previously mentioned baseline assessments, this may not be necessary and may not be available from all health service providers.

Exercise prescription for CHF

As with rehabilitation for any other cardiac population, an individualised exercise training programme should be applied (Myers, 2008; Piña et al., 2003; SIGN, 2002). Following the pre-training assessment, the exercise prescription should be tailored to each person's pathophysiological, psychosocial and vocational needs and tailored to their physical activity preferences and goals (Myers, 2008). As outlined by Lang and Mancini (2007), cognitive impairment is common amongst the CHF population and needs to be considered in the organisation of the exercise programme. An abnormal prevalence of cognitive dysfunction ranging from 35% to more than 50% has been described among patients with CHF. Reduced cardiac output from CHF may further compromise cerebral blood flow in a patient with borderline perfusion of the cerebrum. Additionally, CHF is largely driven by vascular disease, and cerebrovascular disease is an important contributor to multi-infarct dementia. At present, no interventions are yet known to improve cognitive performance, largely because of incomplete knowledge about the pathophysiology of cognitive dysfunction in these patients. Strategies in the exercise class to help with cognitive dysfunction include the following:

- Large circuit boards with pictures
- Simple class set-up with continuous reminders of levels etc.
- Stickers with names for impaired memory
- Reinforcement of key points during class, for example during warm-up; one such key point may be 'what muscle are we stretching?'

Importantly, exercise training for CHF should sufficiently stimulate peripheral skeletal muscles without significantly centrally loading the cardiovascular system, as excessive central stress may be detrimental to left ventricular functioning (ESC, 2001). The programme can incorporate aerobic and strength training, and an interval training approach is widely recommended, especially where baseline exercise tolerance is low (ACPICR, 2006).

The following parameters must be established prior to exercise: mode, duration of each training session, exercise intensity, frequency and programme length (i.e. FITT principle), along with appropriate warm-up and cool-down periods (see section 'Safety and Monitoring'). As people with CHF may experience 'good' and 'bad' days, in terms of symptomatic limitation and overall feeling of well-being, exercise prescription must be flexible, as it may have to be modified from session to session.

Use of interval training in CHF

The basic principle of interval training is to use short bouts of exercise interspersed with lower paced periods (active recovery phase) of similar or longer duration (ACSM, 2006). For people with a low level of baseline exercise tolerance, interval training may be better tolerated initially than steady-state training (Meyer *et al.*, 1996; Thow, 2006). As exercise capacity increases, work phase intensity may be increased, or active recovery phases shortened, in relation to work phases for continued training gains. Interval training enables application of a more intense exercise stimulus on peripheral muscles than may be obtained during steady-state training, and thus produces a more pronounced training effect (Wisløff *et al.*, 2007). Excessive left ventricular stress is avoided, as active recovery phases delay central cardiovascular responses (Meyer *et al.*, 2004).

For aerobic interval training, ESC (2001) suggests that combining initial work phases of 30 seconds with recovery phases of 60 seconds may be practical when used with a work phase intensity of 50% of maximum short-term exercise capacity. Although other combinations, such as 15 seconds work/60 seconds recovery and 10 seconds work/60 seconds recovery, using work phases set at 70–80% maximum exercise capacity have also proved to be effective (Meyer *et al.*, 1996), patients may not comfortably tolerate this intensity, thus limiting their exercise enjoyment. Careful consideration should be given if using training to such a high proportion of maximum capacity. This may be confusing in relation to advice given regarding the pace of physical activity undertaken outside the training programme. Using a baseline exercise test to determine the load for work periods will ensure that exercise is safe and appropriate for the person (Meyer *et al.*, 2004). Further discussion on training intensity is provided later in section 'Exercise Intensity and Pacing for CHF'.

Aerobic training modes for CHF

When selecting training modality or discussing a chosen activity with a person, it may be useful to consider the following:
• Has its safety as a training modality for people with CHF been confirmed by research?
• Is it able to provide a low workload for people with severe exercise intolerance?
• Is it amenable to an interval training protocol?

• Can small and short exercise increments be applied to it (for interval training and to allow training to be gradually progressed)?
• Is the exercise functional and will the training effect transfer to daily activity?

Cycling for CHF

Research has evaluated the efficacy of aerobic training modalities for this population, most commonly focusing on cycling ergometry. Cycling is ideal for applying interval training, and the nature of cycling appropriately stresses peripheral muscles without causing excessive central cardiovascular stress (ESC, 2001). Cycle ergometry is advisable for people with severe exercise intolerance, allowing exercise at very low workloads and reproducibility of a prescribed or tolerated external workload (ESC, 2001). For those who require close observation of cardiovascular exercise responses, cycling allows close monitoring of heart rate and blood pressure during training and may thus be the safest exercise option. For people who have comorbidities, meaning that they are unable to satisfactorily complete weight-bearing activity sufficient to elicit a conditioning response (e.g. osteoarthritis), cycling may provide an appropriate alternative (Thow, 2006). However, as with any modality that relies on specific exercise training equipment, if cycling does not feature in the participant's daily life, the activity is not particularly functional.

Smart *et al.* (2003) state that outdoor cycling may be difficult to pace and, added environmental factors, for example headwinds, cold temperature or a small incline, may require effort in excess of the exercise capacity of the person. Environmental factors have to be considered when prescribing any outdoor programme for this symptomatically limited patient group. For those who are anxious or underconfident about managing their symptomatic limitations during exercise, supervised indoor activity may be preferable until they feel confident about exercising autonomously. Furthermore, it is difficult (and expensive) to closely monitor haemodynamic responses to outdoor activities for those who require close supervision (Smart *et al.*, 2003). Consequently, outdoor activities may be best for those who have been stable in the longer term and who have a good baseline exercise capacity (>5 metabolic equivalents or METs).

Walking for CHF

Although outdoor walking may be well tolerated by the majority of patients, little research has been conducted to establish its efficacy as a training mode for people with CHF. Adherence to home walking programmes can be variable and is difficult to monitor. However, walking does not require any equipment and is functional and inexpensive. Whilst treadmill walking may be easier to pace and amenable to both interval training and close monitoring of exercise responses (Smart *et al.*, 2003), walking on level ground may be better tolerated, particularly by frail and/or elderly people likely to be intimidated by treadmill equipment. As a speed of 80 m/min is the lowest that allows a comfortable jogging movement, it is generally not advisable for people with CHF (Smart *et al.*, 2003), as even this low level requires a reasonable level of exercise tolerance (7 METs).

Water-based activity for CHF

The safety and appropriateness of water-based exercise therapy for people with CHF has been questioned (ESC, 2001). In people with NYHA class III CHF, Meyer and Bűcking (2004) found that immersion in water to neck level resulted in abnormal cardiac responses. These included left ventricular overload and an inability of stroke volume to increase appropriately, thus increasing the risk of further ventricular dilation. Meyer and Bűcking (2004) state that relatively high central haemodynamic stress may occur even during slow- or moderate-paced swimming and highlight that the physiologic requirement of swimming at slow speeds is similar to more vigorously paced dry-land activity. Swimming at a leisurely pace exerts the same physiological effect as cycle ergometry at 100–150 W (approximately 7 METs), and thus may exceed the exercise capacity of many people with CHF (ESC, 2001).

Decompensated CHF is an absolute contraindication for immersion in water and swimming (Meyer and Bűcking, 2004). Therapeutic water exercises (e.g. for orthopaedic reasons) can be allowed for people with NYHA class III CHF, provided the individual remains upright and is immersed maximally to the base of the sternum. Meyer and Bűcking (2004) state that further studies on the safety of swimming and aqua-aerobics are required, and SIGN (2007a) recommends that for individuals of NYHA class III or IV, other forms of physical activity are preferable to exercises in water or swimming.

Circuit stations for CHF

In cardiac rehabilitation, circuits are a popular method of delivering structured exercise sessions (Thow, 2006). Simple aerobic exercise stations (i.e. work phases) positioned around the exercise area (interspersed with active recovery exercise) can effectively provide interval training. The circuit may be designed with minimal equipment, and exercises can be tailored to suit individual's daily activities, thus making them functional. Circuits offer variety, and each station can be adapted to allow for individual's ability, for example arm movements added or removed to increase or reduce work (Thow, 2006). They also facilitate social interaction during exercise, and allow close monitoring of participants by the exercise leader who can circulate around the room and provide individual guidance/assistance where required (Thow, 2006). As they require minimal equipment, circuits can be used to form the basis of a home exercise programme. The use of CDs, videos and Physiotools (2005) can be an effective way to provide home exercise programmes for this group. Thow (2006) provides further

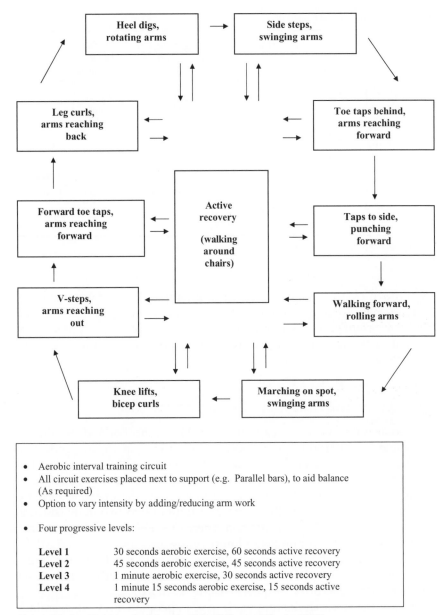

Figure 3.2 Aerobic interval training circuit for CHF group (Cowie, 2008).

guidance on the use of circuits and circuit design. See Figure 3.2 for an example of an interval circuit used for CHF (Cowie, 2008).

For people with severe deconditioning (<3 METs), a seated or standing programme of simple upper and lower limb exercises, for example hip flexion/extension/abduction and knee flexion/extension, may be sufficient

Table 3.2 Aerobic training modalities.

Mode	Safe	Low loads	Small and short increments	Interval training possible	Functional
Cycle ergometry	✓	✓	✓	✓	×
Treadmill	✓		✓	Usually	Usually	×
Outdoor walking	✓		✓	✓	✓	✓
Outdoor cycling	Depends on exercise capacity	×	Possibly	✓	Possibly
Jogging	Unsure	×	✓	✓	Possibly
Swimming	Not confirmed	×	Possibly	Possibly	Possibly
Circuits (interval training)	If appropriately designed (see Figure 3.2)	✓	✓	✓	✓

Adapted from Smart *et al.* (2003).

to improve exercise tolerance. Repeating simple functional movements that mimic those used in a typical muscle-strengthening programme, at a low, comfortable pace, without resistance, may improve endurance during daily activities. Table 3.2 provides an evaluation of training modalities (Smart *et al.*, 2003).

Frequency and duration of exercise for CHF

For people with an exercise capacity of <3 METs, short periods (lasting 5–10 minutes), with multiple daily sessions of activity, are the most effective and best-tolerated forms of exercise (ESC, 2001). For those who develop exhaustion after training, a day of rest between sessions may be required (Piña *et al.*, 2003). As exercise tolerance increases, the duration of daily sessions should be gradually lengthened until one to two daily sessions lasting for 15 minutes can be attained. Thereafter, ESC (2001) suggests that as exercise capacity continues to improve towards and beyond 5 METs, exercise duration should be gradually increased to meet the 30-minute, five times per week physical activity recommendation advocated for all adults to minimise cardiovascular risk (SIGN, 2007b).

Most of the research relating to exercise in people with CHF examines exercise sessions of 20–30 minutes' duration, and ESC (2001) highlights that for those with a good exercise capacity (≥5 METs), this duration will achieve physical and psychosocial benefits. In this fitter functional group, structured, supervised exercise sessions should be supplemented with home exercise to ensure that the desired frequency (five times per week) is achieved (Piña *et al.*, 2003).

Exercise intensity and pacing for CHF

Exercise intensity should be sufficient for physiological gains, tailored to baseline exercise capacity and set at a safe level (Thow, 2006). Training intensities that are too high may cause ischaemia or arrhythmia and increase risk of exercise-related cardiac events. Only those intensities that are tolerated symptom free during baseline exercise testing can be safely prescribed (Meyer et al., 2004). Furthermore, to maximise psychological training gains, the prescribed intensity should be perceived as achievable and enjoyable by the person (Thow, 2006). In CHF, exercise intensity is most commonly described either as a percentage of peak oxygen uptake (pVO$_2$), peak heart rate (PHR), heart rate reserve (HRR/Karvonen formula) or as rating of perceived exertion (RPE) (Borg, 1998).

In terms of pVO$_2$, research has most commonly evaluated training programmes that mimic workloads equating to 60–70% pVO$_2$, as measured during a symptom-limited baseline metabolic exercise test. If this workload cannot be replicated within the exercise session, the heart rate observed during the test for this percentage of pVO$_2$ can be used instead to guide intensity. Exercise intensities of 70% or above pVO$_2$ have been examined with this population and have proved to be safe and successful. The objective of applying such high exercise intensity is to prioritise skeletal muscle or peripheral blood vessel adaptations. However, this can only be applied for short periods, that is, during short work phases as part of interval training (Smart et al., 2003).

For people who are more debilitated, lower intensities (40–60% pVO$_2$) may be more appropriate, and individuals with very poor exercise tolerance will initially best respond to lower exercise intensity (Myers, 2008). Importantly, evidence suggests that exercise intensity does not seem to influence directly the magnitude of gain in exercise tolerance (Meyer et al., 1997b). Moreover, because intensity and duration of exercise session are closely interrelated in terms of training gain, low exercise intensity can be partly compensated for by higher frequency of sessions (in less fit individuals) or longer duration (in people with the capacity for endurance, but not higher intensity). In people who are debilitated, exercise intensity can be increased from 40 to 60% pVO$_2$ when exercise duration of 15 minutes can be achieved (ACPICR, 2006).

Often cardiac rehabilitation programmes do not have access to metabolic exercise testing (i.e. a measure of pVO$_2$) for use as exercise prescription. Because of its relatively linear relationship with pVO$_2$, the heart rate obtained during baseline exercise testing is often used instead (ACSM, 2006). Although ESC (2001) states that training heart rate should be kept as low as possible (where exercise sufficiently stimulates the periphery with minimal central cardiovascular stress), intensities of 40–80% HRR and 60–80% PHR have successfully been applied (ACPICR, 2006). ACSM (2006) and ACPICR (2006) provide explanations for determining the HRR training method. Using PHR obtained from a baseline exercise test is more accurate than using age-predicted maximum heart rate in exercise prescription calculations. This is because the high incidence of arrhythmia and widespread use of chronotropic medications in this population causes the heart rate to deviate from 'normal' age-predicted values. In addition, for safety, heart rate thresholds for internal defibrillators and pacemakers should be identified pre-training and taken into consideration when prescribing training heart rates (ACPICR, 2006) (see Chapter 5).

Piña *et al.* (2003) state that heart rate-derived exercise prescriptions may be inaccurate in people with more advanced disease. As CHF progresses, chronic overstimulation of the sympathetic nervous system eventually limits chronotropic reserve, that is, resting heart rate is higher, and has less capacity to increase during exercise. Furthermore, because people with CHF frequently have pacemakers inserted, and ectopy or atrial fibrillation done, heart rate measurement can be difficult and often inaccurate (Smart *et al.*, 2003). Ratings of exertion (Borg, 1998) are therefore considered an important adjunct to monitoring training responses (ESC, 2001). For individuals typically limited by dyspnoea and/or fatigue, using exertion ratings will help them to recognise exercise responses and gain knowledge and confidence in relation to appropriate self-pacing during activity. Ability to self-pace during training may then transfer to daily activity (Thow, 2006).

Rating of perceived exertion for CHF

Borg (1998) devised two scales of perceived exertion: the 6–20 RPE and the category ratio 10-point scale (CR-10). The RPE was devised first and designed to relate closely to pVO_2 and PHR (Thow, 2006). Whilst the CR-10 scale is most appropriate for identifying one particular sensation during exercise, the RPE (6–20) enables individuals to give an overall rating of how they feel. For submaximal exercise, Thow (2006) advocates use of the RPE (6–20), as both muscle and breathing sensations respond in an almost linear fashion to a submaximal exercise stimulus. Therefore, a person can easily give an overall rating of how they feel.

Thow (2006) states that the CR-10 may be the preferred scale for people limited predominantly by dyspnoea (i.e. limited by one overriding sensation). The ESC (2001) states that people with CHF should rate fatigue and dyspnoea separately during exercise, as the two symptoms are often perceived differently. Essentially, the accuracy of either scale is dependent on careful demonstration by the exercise leader to ensure appropriate use throughout the training programme. (Further guidance on this is provided by Borg, 1998, and Thow, 2006, Ch. 3.) Whichever scale is used, an RPE of 12–13 or CR-10 rating of 3–4 is usually well tolerated by people who have stable CHF (ESC, 2001; Piña *et al.*, 2003).

Metabolic levels of activities for CHF

Ainsworth *et al.* (2000) provide an updated list of the intensity/metabolic requirement of many different recreational, occupational and household activities. Although only estimated values, the MET level required for a particular activity on the list may be compared to that obtained from a recent exercise test, and is thus used to advise people on the suitability of undertaking their chosen activity (Ainsworth *et al.*, 2000). If the activity is vital to an individual's daily function, but it appears to be in excess of their physical capability, it may be possible to suggest ways to lessen its metabolic requirement (e.g. reduce arm work or perform while sitting). For those with severe exercise intolerance, advice on energy conservation techniques (e.g. prioritise tasks and divide into manageable segments, with rests between) may also be useful. Although little research has been done to evaluate the use of energy conservation for people with CHF, there is evidence to confirm its effectiveness with other clinical populations (e.g. chronic obstructive pulmonary disease) who have similar symptoms to CHF (Velloso and Jardim, 2006).

Progression and duration of programme for CHF

The CHF exercise programmes evaluated in the literature vary considerably in terms of duration. Studies have elicited physical and psychosocial gains from programmes lasting between 8 weeks and 1 year. With less evidence to support the use of longer term programmes, more research in this area is currently required (Rees *et al.*, 2004). Piña *et al.* (2003) stress that training programmes should be designed to allow rehabilitation staff to adjust and progress the exercise prescription for continued training gains, as participant's exercise tolerance increases. Although progression of the programme should be tailored to suit baseline exercise capacity, clinical status, adaptability to the programme and comorbidities, ESC (2001) suggests that exercise training should be delivered and progressed in three stages: 'initial', 'improvement' and 'maintenance'.

For people with low baseline exercise tolerance, an 'initial' stage of training at an exercise intensity of 40–50% pVO_2 is advocated. It is recommended that this stage not last longer than 4 weeks, and duration and frequency of training should be increased according to symptoms and clinical status until an exercise duration of 10–15 minutes can be achieved. Meyer *et al.* (1997a) state that people with a low baseline exercise capacity will demonstrate faster and more pronounced adaptation to exercise training during this period than those with a higher capacity.

The primary aim of the next 'improvement' stage is to gradually increase exercise intensity and then to lengthen the exercise session to 15–20 minutes (30 minutes if possible) over 16–26 weeks. ESC (2001) states that beyond this 6-month improvement stage, the exercise programme should be continued to sustain training gains in the 'maintenance' stage. This progression and duration of exercise training is advocated because it is suggested that the maximum time required to attain peak physiological responses and gains is between 16 and 26 weeks. Thereafter, responses plateau (ESC, 2001).

Muscle endurance and strength training for CHF

Although exercise programmes frequently focus on exercise to improve aerobic capacity, strength and flexibility are also important components of fitness (Graves and Franklin, 2001). Importantly, strengthening skeletal muscles may reverse the loss of skeletal muscle volume and strength, which is characteristic of the normal ageing process and accelerated in CHF (Braith and Beck, 2008).

Historically, there has been a reluctance to incorporate resistance/ strengthening exercise into CHF training, based on potentially harmful cardiovascular responses elicited during isometric sustained grip exercises in various studies in the 1980s (ESC, 2001). Although the safety of resistance training in people with CHF needs to be further established in large trials, several recent studies have demonstrated that clinical improvement can be safely attained from dynamic isotonic training that is focused on improving skeletal muscle endurance, rather than maximal strength (Meyer *et al.*, 2004). Importantly, improving muscle endurance will enhance the ability to perform repeated muscle actions against submaximal resistance, as is required during daily activity.

Braith and Beck (2008) have outlined absolute and relative contraindications specific to resistance training for people with CHF classified as NYHA class I, II or III (Table 3.3), many of which are similar to those outlined by ESC (2001) (Table 3.2). Importantly, the authors highlight that due to lack of available evidence to date, NYHA class IV is currently considered an absolute contraindication to resistance training. Essentially, for people

Table 3.3 Contraindications to resistance training in chronic heart failure.

Relative contraindications	Absolute contraindications
Unstable angina pectoris	NYHA classification IV
New onset of atrial fibrillation	Obstruction of left ventricular outflow
Severe pulmonary hypertension	Decompensated CHF
Complex ventricular arrhythmias at rest	Threatening arrhythmias
Arrhythmias which increase in severity/ frequency with exercise	Exercise capacity of ≤ 3 METs Moderate-to-severe aortic stenosis
Significant exercise-induced ischaemia (>3 mm ST segment depression)	Uncontrolled diabetes

Braith and Beck (2008).

classified as NYHA class IV, simple, repeated, unresisted limb movements may be sufficient to improve skeletal muscle strength.

Generally, rhythmic exercise, alternating between opposing small muscle groups to prevent overtiring of one muscle group, is recommended for people with CHF (ACPICR, 2006). Konstantinos and Tokmakidis (2005) state that, based on available evidence, people of only CHF NYHA class I can perform whole-body (bilateral) resistance exercises; those of NYHA class II and class III should be advised only on segmental (unilateral) resistance exercise.

The upper limb muscles tend to be neglected in training programmes. However, they should not be ignored because many daily activities require arm work (Piña *et al.*, 2003). As people with CHF are more likely to experience fatigue and dyspnoea during upper, rather than lower, body activity, they may typically restrict use of their arms and the upper limb muscles are likely to become deconditioned. Protracted posture of the shoulder girdle and use of accessory muscles for breathing may occur; hence, the importance of maintaining good posture during muscle endurance exercises should be emphasised (ACPICR, 2006).

As with other cardiac populations, sustained isometric exercises that involve breath holding and Valsalva manoeuvre should be avoided, due to the associated rapid increase in rate pressure product, which significantly increases myocardial oxygen demand and hence the risk of cardiac ischaemia and arrhythmia (Braith and Beck, 2008). During seated activity and/or upper limb activity, the feet should be kept moving to maintain venous return and cardiac output (ACPICR, 2006).

Emphasis should be placed on low weights and high repetitions, with short work phases, especially initially and during seated exercise (ACPICR, 2006). The ACPICR (2006) suggests that a suitable programme of muscle strength and endurance training for people with CHF may incorporate 8–10 exercise stations, each involving the performance of 1 set of 10–15 repetitions. More recently, Braith and Beck (2008) outlined more specific recommendations and highlighted that resistance training parameters should be tailored and progressed according to any improvement in NYHA classification. As shown in Table 3.4, they suggest that 3–9 resistance exercise stations are used, each involving the performance of 1–3 sets of 4–15 repetitions for each activity.

A work recovery ratio of 1:2 for muscle strength and endurance is recommended by the ESC (2001), ACPICR (2006) and Braith and Beck (2008). Thow (2006) recommends that recovery periods should not exceed 1 minute; otherwise endurance benefits may be reduced. Perceived exertion ratings may be used to guide intensity. ESC (2001) recommends an RPE <13 (3–4 on CR-10) for muscle strength and endurance training, whilst Braith and Beck (2008) advocate a similar RPE of 11–14 (2.5–5.0 on CR-10).

The ACPICR (2006) and Braith and Beck (2008) indicate that the weight or resistance should equate to approximately 40–60% of one 'repetition

Table 3.4 Recommendations for resistance training for people with chronic heart failure.

Characteristic	NYHA class I	NYHA classes II–III
Frequency	2–3 days/week	1–2 days/week
Intensity	50–60% 1RM	40–50% 1RM
Work/recovery ratio	≥1:2	≥1:2
Number of exercise stations	4–9	3–4
Number of sets per station	2–3	1–2
Number of repetitions per set	6–15	4–10

Braith and Beck (2008).

maximum' (1RM) (the maximum weight that can be lifted by an individual in one smooth, continuous movement). However, ascertaining a baseline 1RM using maximal workloads can lead to Valsalva and other cardiovascular complications and is not recommended for any cardiac population (Thow, 2006). For people with CHF, low resistant loads should be used initially and increased gradually throughout the programme as considered appropriate. Performing exercises without resistance to ensure correct, safe technique may be most prudent initially. The appropriate duration for this 'resistance-free' period has not yet been established and should be based on the person's ability to establish the correct technique and response to training.

Whilst Braith and Beck (2008) advise that training frequency is progressed from once to three times per week (Table 3.4), ACPICR (2006) states that muscle strength and endurance training should be performed two to three times per week for optimal training gains. The ACPICR (2006) indicates that this may be incorporated into the aerobic component of a training programme, interspersed between aerobic stations to provide active recovery stations in an interval circuit and using an aerobic (work phase) muscle endurance (active recovery phase) ratio of 1:1 or 2:1. Braith and Beck (2008) and Smart *et al.* (2003) highlight that various authors have demonstrated that combining aerobic and resistance training in CHF rehabilitation is more effective than using each training method separately.

Available evidence indicates that improvements in strength and endurance may occur after 4–6 weeks of training (Smart *et al.*, 2003). Currently, there is a lack of evidence to suggest an optimal duration for an endurance and strength training programme, or whether training gains are maintained in the longer term after programme cessation.

Exercise to improve flexibility and coordination for CHF

At present, in the absence of substantial supporting evidence, training consisting of coordination and flexibility has been suggested to be of value in people with CHF (Meyer *et al.*, 2004). In particular, fatigue and dyspnoea associated with arm and upper body exercise can lead to poor posture and use of accessory muscles for breathing, causing maladaptations of structure and function of the soft tissues of the upper body (ACPICR, 2006). Subsequently, exercises designed to improve posture, flexibility and coordination may enhance performance of daily tasks, and may be incorporated into components of an aerobic and strengthening programme or undertaken separately. As these exercises have a low cardiovascular load they are unlikely to increase health risks beyond those of endurance training (Meyer *et al.*, 2004).

Safety and monitoring

Patient safety during exercise is paramount (Boudreau and Genovese, 2007). Smart and Marwick (2004) evaluated 64 CHF exercise training studies and found no deaths directly attributable to exercise in more than 59 000 patient-hours. Indeed, provided exercise is appropriately prescribed, there is little evidence that exercise worsens left ventricular function or increases heart chamber size (Stewart *et al.*, 2003). However, although adverse effects directly relating to exercise are infrequent, people are susceptible to complications because of their left ventricular dysfunction and overactive sympathetic nervous system (Stewart *et al.*, 2003). Furthermore, in a population in which functional class often changes, it is difficult to ascertain whether worsening symptoms are due to the variability of CHF or due to exercise (Piña *et al.*, 2003). Consequently, members of the rehabilitation team should be skilled in monitoring this population during exercise and should provide an appropriate level of supervision of all individuals during exercise sessions (ACPICR, 2006).

For structured exercise rehabilitation, the ACPICR (2006) recommends that patient/staff ratio ranges from 3:1 to 5:1 depending on the overall risk stratification of the individuals attending the programme at any time. People who are very physically limited by CHF or other comorbidities may require 1:1 supervision or assistance with exercise, which may restrict class size if staffing resources are limited. Exercise attendance may be erratic, as a person may have a 'bad' day in terms of symptom limitation and decide that a day of rest and energy conservation is more appropriate than exercising.

Home exercise programmes and behaviour change for CHF
Historically, the belief that people with CHF require close supervision during exercise has meant that research has predominantly focused on supervised and/or hospital-based training. Home-based training may, however, offer a more pragmatic rehabilitation option for people limited by CHF (Smart and Marwick, 2004). Exercising at home does not involve a potentially tiring journey to a hospital, and in contrast to scheduled hospital sessions, it can be undertaken at a time of day when the person feels most

able to exercise (due to their physical or motivational state or daily commitments). Home programmes can be devised using many formats, for example DVDs, videos and Physiotools; these programmes can be replicas of the hospital-based classes (Cowie, 2008). The patient can carry out the exercise at home when it best suits them. Motivational interviewing to enhance motivation and behaviour change (i.e. adoption of physical activity) has been found to enhance adherence and outcomes from an entirely home exercise programme in people with CHF (Brodie and Inoue, 2005). Thereafter, frequent follow-up (e.g. by telephone or review appointments) could then provide means of monitoring and progressing a home-based programme and resolving any exercise-related problems (Piña *et al.*, 2003) (see Thow, 2006, Ch. 8, for more on motivational interviewing).

Conversely, the benefits of social interaction associated with supervised group exercise are well documented, and as feelings of depression and social isolation are common within the CHF population, psychosocial benefits may be limited from a home programme undertaken without peer support (Berry and McMurray, 1999). Combining supervised and unsupervised exercise training may boost confidence during exercise, thus facilitating adherence to the exercise prescription, particularly in the longer term, when the person is able to progress to independent exercise (Smart *et al.*, 2003). Currently, with insufficient evidence to confirm the safety or efficacy of exercise as entirely home based, an initial period of supervised exercise is recommended by many authors for people with CHF (Piña *et al.*, 2003). Intermittent sessions of unsupervised exercise training may be added to the supervised sessions when the person is clinically stable, can safely exercise within the prescribed training range and feels ready to exercise independently.

In terms of safety, the initial period of supervision during exercise allows prompt identification of signs or symptoms, indicating the need to modify or terminate an exercise session (Boudreau and Genovese, 2007). Prior to each session, Smart *et al.* (2003) recommend that symptoms, body weight and any peripheral oedema are assessed. Pre- and post-exercise resting heart rate and blood pressure should also be measured. Such measurements will ensure a person's suitability to participate in the exercise session, and may help to reveal subtle signs and symptoms that commonly precede clinical decompensation and, with prompt intervention, could avert hospitalisation (Stewart *et al.*, 2003).

The most common exercise-related complications are post-exercise hypotension, atrial and ventricular arrhythmias, and worsening symptoms, indicating that people with arrhythmias and those with more advanced CHF should be closely monitored during training (Piña *et al.*, 2003). The ESC (2001) advocates use of telemetry during initial exercise sessions. However, this may be unrealistic for some health providers and unnecessary if cardiac symptoms, heart rate and RPE are closely monitored. Recommendations in relation to this issue are varied, and acknowledging that telemetry is expensive, Myers (2008) indicates that only a small percentage of people with more advanced CHF require continuous telemetry during exercise.

Warm-up and cool-down for CHF

Each period of exercise should be preceded by a warm-up session and concluded with a cool-down session. For a 20- to 30-minute exercise session, the warm-up and cool-down periods should each last at least 15 minutes, as they are essential for decreasing the likelihood of cardiovascular complications that may occur at the onset or recovery phases of exercise (Piña *et al.*, 2003). The warm-up period facilitates optimal coronary vasodilation to prepare the myocardium for exercise, while the cool-down phase prevents pooling of blood in extremities and maintains venous return (and thus cardiac output) during recovery (ACSM, 2006). Without these appropriately timed transition periods, people with CHF are at particular risk of cardiac ischaemia, post-exercise hypotension or ventricular dysrhythmias (ACPICR, 2006). Furthermore, people should ideally be closely monitored for up to 30 minutes in the immediate post-exercise period, that is, for a further 15 minutes after the cool-down period.

Prolonged warm-up and cool-down periods are inappropriate for people with extremely poor exercise tolerance, for example <3 METs. This group will have been prescribed a training programme of short, multiple daily exercise sessions at a low intensity, and shorter warm-up and cool-down periods are recommended.

The exercise session should be terminated if an acute decrease in blood pressure, or sudden onset of angina, significant dyspnoea fatigue and/or serious exercise-induced rhythm disorders are observed, or if any other contraindication to exercise training develops (ESC, 2001). In this instance appropriate medical review should be sought, and the person should return to the training programme when clinical stability is restored, for example when arrhythmias or symptoms have been fully investigated and optimally managed (Smart *et al.*, 2003).

Medication issues for CHF

People with CHF may be prescribed multi-pharmacology, composed of cardiac and non-cardiac medication. An awareness of the exercise-related issues surrounding the three main cardiac medications is important for rehabilitation staff involved in delivering and monitoring exercise for this population.

Angiotensin-converting enzyme inhibitors for CHF

All people with CHF should be considered for angiotensin-converting enzyme (ACE) inhibitor medication unless contraindicated by a history of renovascular impairment or angioedema (ESC, 2005; NICE, 2003;

SIGN, 2007a). ACE inhibitors have been found to reduce hospital admissions, due to worsening CHF by 27% and a relative risk of mortality by 26% (Flather *et al.*, 2000). People may experience an improvement in their CHF symptoms within a few weeks or few months after commencing ACE inhibitor use (SIGN, 2007a).

Due to their antihypertensive activity, ACE inhibitors may cause symptomatic/asymptomatic hypotension when first taken or when the medication is uptitrated to an optimum dose (ESC, 2005; SIGN, 2007a). Throughout the training programme, staff should enquire of patients and participants should inform rehabilitation staff of any planned changes to medication doses. Pre- and post-exercise measurement of blood pressure will identify hypotension, and it is prudent to advise people to avoid exercise on the day when an increased dose is taken for the first time. Generally, asymptomatic hypotension does not require any change in therapy, though if people present with associated dizziness, light-headedness and/or confusion, they should avoid exercise and be advised to consult the appropriate health care professional (heart failure nurse or doctor) regarding revising the medication (NICE, 2003; SIGN, 2007a).

Cough is another side effect of ACE inhibitor medication. A persistent, troublesome, dry cough may eventually warrant a change in medication. However, those presenting with a 'new' cough should be fully assessed to exclude the possibility of pulmonary oedema, that is, onset of decompensation (NICE, 2003; SIGN, 2007a). People intending to prevent/alleviate aggravation of long-standing musculoskeletal discomfort during exercise with non-steroidal anti-inflammatory drugs (NSAIDs) should be advised to avoid those not prescribed by a doctor due to risk of interaction with ACE inhibitors (SIGN, 2007a).

β-Blockade therapy for CHF

β-Blockers also improve morbidity and mortality associated with CHF, reducing mortality caused by cardiac pump failure by 36% (Domanksi *et al.*, 2003). β-Blockers are contraindicated in those with asthma, heart block (<60 beats/min) or symptomatic hypotension (SIGN, 2007a). The clinical state should be stable before the drug is commenced, and symptomatic improvement is likely after 3–6 months (NICE, 2003).

Once initiated, β-blockers are uptitrated very gradually to target doses, as patients can experience temporary symptomatic deterioration and decompensation during initiation or uptitration (ESC, 2005; NICE, 2003; SIGN, 2007a). Thus, as with ACE inhibitors, staff should enquire of patients and patients should keep rehabilitation staff informed of any impending change in dosage whilst they are participating in a training programme. They can continue to exercise during initiation or uptitration, but should vigilantly monitor body weight, oedema, dyspnoea and fatigue, and report any worsening symptoms to staff (NICE, 2003; SIGN, 2007a). Those presenting with worsening symptoms or signs of decompensation should abstain from exercise and be promptly referred to the appropriate health care professional for review of medication. As with ACE inhibitors, β-blockers can also cause hypotension. Again, this does not usually necessitate withdrawal of the drug unless the person becomes symptomatic (NICE, 2003; SIGN, 2007a).

As β-blockers lower heart rate, this should be taken into consideration when prescribing training heart rates for patients. Importantly, if resting heart rate falls below 50 beats/min, the medication dose may require to be reduced. Identification of such bradycardia at an exercise session requires appropriate review (SIGN, 2007a).

Diuretics with CHF

People with CHF may be considered for diuretic therapy if they suffer from dyspnoea or oedema (peripheral or pulmonary) (ESC, 2005; SIGN, 2007a). Diuretics can reduce mortality in those with CHF by 75% and improve exercise capacity by 63% (Faris *et al.*, 2002). After taking diuretic medication, a person may spend a considerable amount of time urinating and may therefore prefer not to attend appointments/exercise sessions until this period has passed. To avoid this situation, they can be advised to alter the timings of taking the diuretics, provided that they are not taken after 6 p.m. (as this may cause nocturia). Furthermore, when encouraging people to remain hydrated during exercise, those taking diuretics may have been advised to restrict their fluid intake (to avoid overload), so they should take only small amounts of fluids. Finally, arthritic gout (accumulation of uric acid) in joints can develop secondary to diuretic medication and can restrict exercise ability. These people should avoid taking NSAIDs not prescribed by a doctor (SIGN, 2007a).

Outcome measures for CHF

Measurement of exercise capacity

In any person with cardiac disease, his or her exercise capacity is an important prognostic indicator (Thow, 2006). Exercise testing is therefore essential pre-training in providing further assessment of the exercise-related risk associated with the higher risk CHF patient group. Furthermore, it allows training to be tailored to any physical capabilities and limitations which become apparent during the test (Mears, 2006).

Measurement of pVO_2 obtained by metabolic cardiopulmonary exercise test is considered the most accurate measure of cardiorespiratory fitness in any individual with symptomatic disease (ACSM, 2006; Ingle, 2007). pVO_2 can be reduced by 50% in people with CHF, and it is an important clinical tool for predicting heart failure mortality and prognosis (Ingle, 2007; Piña *et al.*, 2003). Indeed, pVO_2 is considered a better predictor of mortality than are measures of central cardiac function in those with CHF

(Belardinelli *et al.*, 1999). A pVO_2 of <10 mL/kg/min indicates a relatively high-risk individual, with a poor 1-year prognosis, whilst a pVO_2 of >18 mL/kg/min categorises a lower risk individual (Ingle, 2007).

Although ESC (2001) advocates obtaining a measure of pre-training pVO_2 to fully assess patient risk and to allow accurate exercise prescription, cardiopulmonary metabolic exercise testing is time-consuming, costly and poorly tolerated by patients (Arnott, 1997). As with other cardiac patient groups, the 6-minute walk test (6 MWT) (Butland *et al.*, 1982) and the incremental shuttle walk test (ISWT) (Singh *et al.*, 1992) have become popular clinical substitutes for cardiopulmonary exercise testing in people with CHF. Field walking tests are inherently simplistic, devoid of equipment, inexpensive and easy to administer (Solway *et al.*, 2001). As walking is familiar to most people, the tests elicit minimal patient anxiety and can be undertaken even by the most severely limited individuals (Singh *et al.*, 1992).

The self-paced 6 MWT is widely used in clinical practice, and its validity and reproducibility have frequently been evaluated (and often confirmed) in relation to CHF and other clinical populations. Solway *et al.* (2001) therefore consider the 6 MWT to be the best test for assessing fitness of individuals suffering from any cardiac or respiratory disease.

Because the test allows people to walk at their own pace, they may not achieve pVO_2 (American Thoracic Society (ATS), 2002). However, the 6 MWT will establish submaximal exercise capacity, which may better reflect ability to undertake daily activity. The 6 MWT may also demonstrate clinically important training gains in relation to submaximal performance, which may have occurred without gains in peak capacity (ATS, 2002). In terms of risk stratification, failure to attain a walking distance of 300 m on the 6 MWT has been associated with poor short-term survival (ACPICR, 2006).

Considering the symptomatic limitations associated with CHF, the self-paced nature of the 6 MWT may allow observation of how patients manage their limitations to enable them to continue with the task, thus aiding exercise prescription (Tobin and Thow, 1999). However, because it is self-paced, the 6 MWT is difficult to standardise, and results may be influenced by patient motivation and therapist encouragement (Guyatt *et al.*, 1984).

The incremental, externally paced ISWT has been found to provide a valid, reproducible measure of pVO_2. However, few trials have been conducted to evaluate its use in CHF. Evidence to support its use with other cardiac patient groups is also generally lacking (Solway *et al.*, 2001).

With its ability to provide a measure of pVO_2, the incremental nature of the ISWT provides a PHR, from which a training heart rate (using HRR) can be set. Furthermore, although the gradual, incremental nature of the ISWT may not reflect daily activity, it may minimise the onset of cardiac symptoms and so may be safer than the 6 MWT (Singh *et al.*, 1992). In addition to being externally paced, the ISWT is easier to standardise than the 6 MWT (Arnott, 1997). However, unlike the 6 MWT, the ISWT may not demonstrate submaximal training effects, particularly in those with poor exercise capacity, as the early exercise levels of the ISWT have been criticised for their lack of sensitivity to change. Essentially, with a lack of consensus on which is the best test, it is for clinicians to decide whether the 6 MWT or the ISWT provides the most useful data, and is most appropriate for their patient group.

Measurement of quality of life in CHF

For people with CHF, quality of life is impaired in many ways. The impairment in physical health, along with a heightened self-awareness of morbidity and mortality, can lead to anxiety and depression. Social activities become curtailed; there is an increased reliance on others and recurrent hospitalisation diminishes autonomy (Berry and McMurray, 1999). In turn, poorer quality of life is associated with higher hospitalisation and mortality (Moser and Worster, 2000). Quality of life is therefore an important treatment outcome, particularly where prognosis is poor and life expectancy limited (Berry and McMurray, 1999). Coelho et al. (2005) highlight that quality of life should be measured pre- and post-training.

Various generic quality-of-life questionnaires have been evaluated for use with CHF: the Medical Outcomes Short Form – 36 (SF-36) (Ware and Sherbourne, 1992), the Sickness Impact Profile (SIP) (Bergener et al., 1976) and the Nottingham Health Profile (NHP) (Hunt et al., 1980). These questionnaires are useful for determining the effects of an intervention on different aspects of quality of life and for comparing data obtained from individuals with one particular medical condition to that obtained from individuals with a different clinical problem (Berry and McMurray, 1999).

The SF-36 is most widely used in clinical practice, and it has been validated for use in CHF (Berry and McMurray, 1999). It can discriminate between heart failure and other medical conditions, and between individuals with heart failure of varying severity (Berry and McMurray, 1999). Some of its questions are, however, considered unsuitable for elderly individuals, thus limiting its application, and there have been reports of floor and ceiling effects when used with other chronic conditions (Dunderdale et al., 2005). However, the SIP and NHP have produced variable results in relation to CHF, and have been criticised for being insensitive to CHF symptoms and to small changes to quality of life (Berry and McMurray, 1999). In addition, while the SIP is time-consuming to complete, the NHP may be too short to provide comprehensive information (Dunderdale et al., 2005). The SF-36 is considered to be of appropriate length and simplicity, and there is consensus that it is the preferred generic questionnaire for use with people with CHF (Berry and McMurray, 1999; Johansson et al., 2004).

Because they provide a broad overview, generic questionnaires may be too insensitive to highlight small changes that are clinically important for one particular group of individuals with one particular medical condition

(Berry and McMurray, 1999). Disease-specific measurement tools can thus provide a more precise assessment of the impact of that condition on an individual's health-related quality of life.

Two questionnaires specific to CHF are the Minnesota Living with Heart Failure Questionnaire (MLHFQ) (Rector *et al.*, 1987) and the Chronic Heart Failure Questionnaire (CHFQ) (Guyatt, 1993). The validity of the MLHFQ is established; it is widely used and it has been found to be sensitive to change (Berry and McMurray, 1999). The MLHFQ can discriminate between those with symptomatic and asymptomatic CHF, but does not distinguish between varying severities (Berry and McMurray, 1999). Concern has been raised regarding its inability to discriminate between factors directly associated with CHF and those associated with an individual's co-morbidities (Dunderdale *et al.*, 2005). The MLHFQ is user friendly, short, easy to administer and easily understood (Berry and McMurray, 1999). The validity of the CHFQ is reasonably established, and it has been found to be sensitive to different severities of CHF and to change elicited by a particular treatment (Berry and McMurray, 1999). However, the CHFQ has to be administered by interview (which is complex) and the literature suggests that more research evaluating its use is required (Dunderdale *et al.*, 2005). Furthermore, whilst generic questionnaires may provide too broad an overview, disease-specific questionnaires may be too specific and too inflexible to take into account factors which do not relate directly to CHF (Guyatt, 1993).

There appears to be no ideal tool for measuring quality of life in people with CHF, as existing questionnaires have their strengths and weaknesses. Many of the questionnaires were designed for research purposes from a health professional's perspective, but not for a person with CHF (Dunderdale *et al.*, 2005). At present, the optimal method for obtaining a comprehensive overview is to use both a generic and a disease-specific questionnaire, though this may be too time-consuming for everyday clinical practice (Berry and McMurray, 1999; Johansson *et al.*, 2004).

Measurement of everyday activity level for CHF

In the general population, physical inactivity increases overall cardiovascular risk (SIGN, 2007b). In CHF, physical impairment restricts the ability to perform normal everyday activities, causing anxiety and fear of movement, leading to more sedentary behaviour. A 'vicious cycle' thus ensues, which is detrimental to physical fitness, quality of life and ultimately prognosis (Van den Berg-Emons *et al.*, 2005). Indeed, Van den Berg-Emons *et al.* (2001) demonstrated that the duration of movement-related daily activities undertaken by people with CHF is considerably lower than that of healthy adults.

Whilst improved exercise capacity through training does not automatically translate to a more active lifestyle, Van den Berg-Emons *et al.* (2004) identified that aerobic training does have the potential to increase daily activity in CHF. Traditionally, health professionals have focused on changes in exercise capacity. However, people who are physically limited by CHF may perceive improvements to daily activity level as more important and relevant (Dunderdale *et al.*, 2005). Measurement of everyday physical activity may be an important treatment outcome in CHF rehabilitation. Currently, few studies have used functional activity levels as a training outcome for CHF.

Verbal reports of habitual physical activity and exercise diaries help rehabilitation staff tailor exercise advice, set training parameters and evaluate rehabilitation outcomes. They can also enhance patient motivation by providing feedback on progress. Although useful, such subjective measures are inaccurate, and there is often discrepancy between what a person says they can do and what they actually do (Oka *et al.*, 1993). Objective measures of everyday physical activity may therefore provide more accurate information.

Although practical, simple and cost-effective, tools such as pedometers and calorimeters only provide information on level of physical activity and no information on the activities performed (Evangelista *et al.*, 2005; Van den Berg-Emons *et al.*, 2005). Van den Berg-Emons *et al.* (2005) used an 'activity monitor' (AM) to measure activity level. The AM provides information on duration, rate and moment of occurrence of daily activities (e.g. lying, sitting, standing, walking and running) over 24 hours, via ambulatory monitoring of signals from accelerometers fixed to the body. However, whilst the AM has been validated for people with CHF (Van den Berg-Emons *et al.*, 2005) and while it can provide detailed data, it may be too expensive and too complicated for routine clinical use. More research in the optimum tool for measuring everyday physical activity level in people with CHF is required.

Key messages

• There will be a significant increase in heart failure sufferers who will be accessing cardiac rehabilitation.
• CHF subjects have many physiological dysfunctions affecting muscle, lung and fluid retention.
• Exercise has considerable benefits on functional activity and quality of life for CHF subjects.
• It is important that the patient daily monitor 'dry' weight (i.e. on waking, after urination and before consumption of any fluid).
• CHF subjects often have cognitive impairment.
• Due to the variability of CHF exercise, professionals need to be flexible in exercise prescription.
• Prolonged warm-up and cool-down is required for CHF.
• Combining aerobic and resistance training in CHF rehabilitation is more effective than using each training method separately.

• The rehabilitation team should be skilled in monitoring this population during exercise and should provide an appropriate level of supervision of CHF subjects during exercise sessions.
• In addition to exercise outcomes quality of life should be measured.
• Exercise-related issues surrounding the three main cardiac medications of ACE inhibitors, β-blockers and diuretics are important for rehabilitation staff involved in delivering and monitoring exercise for this population.

Summary and conclusions

Although the pathophysiological changes of CHF are extensive and complex, a large body of evidence indicates that this population can benefit from participating in a cardiac rehabilitation programme and increasing habitual activity.

However, it remains unclear how physical activity can be promoted in this population over the long term. Encouraging an increase in habitual exercise is one of the main aims of cardiac rehabilitation with this group.

It is crucial that physical activity behaviour changes are maintained, as those with CHF have many barriers to activity and exercise. Cognitive behavioural interventions, such as motivational interviewing, phone calls, group exercise and physical activity consultation, have potential to be effective in the CHF population.

Areas for future research include the organisation and components of exercise training programmes and optimal methods to evaluate the benefits that people with CHF derive from them.

References

Adamopoulos, S., Parissis, J., Karatzas, D., *et al.* (2002) Physical training modulates proinflammatory cytokines and the soluble Fas/soluble Fasligand system in patients with chronic heart failure. *Journal of the American College of Cardiology*, 39, 653–63.

Ainsworth, B.E., Haskell, W.L., Leon, A.S. (2000) Compendium of physical activities: an update of activity codes and MET intensities. *Medicine Science Sport and Exercise*, 32, S498–516.

American Association of Cardiovascular and Pulmonary Rehabilitation (AACVPR) (2006) *Guidelines for Cardiac Rehabilitation and Secondary Prevention Programs*, 5th edn. Champaign, IL: Human Kinetics.

American College of Sports Medicine (ACSM) (2006) *Guidelines for Exercise Testing and Prescription*, 7th edn. Baltimore, MD: Lippincott, Williams & Wilkins.

American Thoracic Society (ATS) (2002) ATS statement: guidelines for the six-minute walk test. *American Journal of Respiratory Critical Care Medicine*, 166, 111–17.

Arnott, A. (1997) Assessment of functional capacity in cardiac rehabilitation. *Coronary Health Care*, 1, 30–36.

Association of Chartered Physiotherapists in Cardiac Rehabilitation (ACPICR) (2006) *Standards for the Exercise Component of Phase III Cardiac Rehabilitation.* London: CSP.

Belardinelli, R. (2003) Arrhythmias during acute and chronic exercise in chronic heart failure. *International Journal of Cardiology*, 90, 213–18.

Belardinelli, R., Georgiou, D., Cianci, G., *et al.* (1999) Randomised, controlled trial of long-term moderate exercise training in chronic heart failure: effects on functional capacity, quality of life and clinical outcome. *Circulation*, 99, 1173–82.

Bergener, M., Bobbitt, R.A., Kressels, S., *et al.* (1976) The sickness impact profile: conceptual formulation and methodology for the development of health status measure. *International Journal of Health Service*, 6, 393–415.

Berry, C., McMurray, J. (1999) A review of quality of life evaluations in patients with congestive heart failure. *Pharmacoeconomics*, 16, 241–71.

Borg, G.A.V. (1998) *Borg's Perceived Exertion and Pain Scales.* Champaign, IL: Human Kinetics.

Boudreau, M. Genovese, J. (2007) Cardiac rehabilitation: a comprehensive program for the management of heart failure. *Progress in Cardiovascular Nursing*, 22, 88–92.

Braith, R.W., Beck, D.T. (2008) Resistance exercise: adaptations and developing a safe exercise prescription. *Heart Failure Reviews*, 13(1), 69–79.

Brodie, D.A., Inoue, A. (2005) Motivational interviewing to promote physical activity for people with chronic heart failure. *Issues and Innovations in Nursing Practice*, 50, 518–27.

Butland, R.J., Pang, J., Gross, E.R. (1982) Two-, six- and 12-minute walking tests in respiratory disease. *British Medical Journal*, 284, 1607–8.

Carson, P., Johnson, G., Fletcher, R., *et al.* (1996) Mild systolic dysfunction in heart failure: baseline characteristics, prognosis and response to therapy in the vasodilator in heart failure trials (V-HeFT). *Journal of the American College of Cardiology*, 27, 642–9.

Chong, A.Y., Lip, G.Y.H. (2007) Viewpoint: the prothrombic state in heart failure. *European Journal of Heart Failure*, 9, 124–8.

Chwan Ng, A.C., Freedman, S.B., Sindone, A.P. (2007) Autonomic abnormalities in congestive heart failure patients with sleep-disordered breathing. *Journal of Cardiac Failure*, 13, 395–400.

Cicoira, M., Maggioni, A.P., Latini, I., *et al.* (2007) Body mass index, prognosis and mode of death in chronic heart failure: results from the Valsartan Heart Failure Trial. *European Journal of Heart Failure*, 9, 397–402.

Coats, A.J., Adamopulos, S., Radaelli, A., *et al.* (1992) Controlled trial of physical training ion chronic heart failure. Exercise performance, haemodynamics, ventilation, and autonomic function. *Circulation*, 85, 2119–31.

Coelho, R., Ramos, S., Prata, J., *et al.* (2005) Heart failure and health related quality of life. *Clinical Practice and Epidemiology in Mental Health*, 1, 1–19.

Cohn, J.N., Johnson, G.R., Shabetai, R., *et al.* (For the V-HeFT VA Cooperative Studies Group) (1993). Ejection fraction, peak exercise oxygen consumption, cardiothoracic ratio, ventricular arrhythmias, and plasma norepinephrine as determinants of prognosis in heart failure. *Circulation*, 87 (Suppl), V15–16.

Conraads, V.M. (2002) Combined endurance/resistance training reduces plasma TNF-alpha receptor levels in patients with chronic heart failure and coronary artery disease. *European Heart Journal*, 23, 1854–60.

Cowie, A. (2008) A *Study Comparing Effects of Home- and Hospital-Based Exercise on Exercise Capacity, Activity Levels and Quality of Life of Patients with Chronic Heart Failure.* Unpublished PhD thesis. Glasgow, UK: Ayrshire and Arran NHS Trust and Glasgow Caledonian University.

Dall'Ago, P., Chiappa, G.R., Guths, H., *et al.* (2006) Inspiratory muscle training in patients with heart failure and inspiratory muscle weakness: a randomized trial. *Journal of the American College of Cardiology*, 47, 757–63.

Das, S.R. (2004) Effects of diabetes mellitus and ischemic heart disease on the progression from asymptomatic left ventricular dysfunction to symptomatic heart failure: a retrospective analysis from the studies of left ventricular dysfunction (SOLVD) prevention trial. *American Heart Journal*, 148, 883–8.

De Keulenaer, G.W., Brutsaert, D.L. (2007) Systolic and diastolic heart failure: different phenotypes of the same disease? *European Journal of Heart Failure*, 9, 136–43.

De Sutter, J.H.A.J., Ascoop, A.K., Van de Veire, N., *et al.* (2005) Exercise training results in a significant reduction in mortality and morbidity in heart failure patients on optimal medical treatment. *European Heart Journal*, 26 (Suppl), Abstract 370.

Department of Health (DH) (2000) *National Service Framework for Coronary Heart Disease.* London: Department of Health.

Domanksi, M.J., Krause-Steinrauf, H., Massie, B.M., *et al.* (2003) A comparative analysis of the results from 4 trials of beta blocker therapy for heart failure: BEST, CIBIS-II, MERIT-HF, and COPERNICUS. *Journal of Cardiac Failure*, 9, 354–63.

Drexler, H., Riede, U., Munzel, T., *et al.* (1992) Alterations of skeletal muscle in chronic heart failure. *Circulation*, 85, 1751–9.

Dunderdale, K., Thompson, D.R., Miles, J.N.V., *et al.* (2005) Quality of life measurement in chronic heart failure: do we take account of the patient perspective? *European Journal of Heart Failure*, 7, 572–82.

European Society of Cardiology (ESC) (2001) Recommendations for exercise training in chronic heart failure patients. *European Heart Journal*, 22, 125–35.

European Society of Cardiology (ESC) (2005) Guidelines for the diagnosis and treatment of chronic heart failure: executive summary (update 2005). *European Heart Journal*, 26, 1115–40.

Evangelista, L., Dracup, K., Erickson, V., *et al.* (2005) Validity of pedometers for measuring exercise adherence in heart failure patients. *Journal of Cardiac Failure*, 11, 366–71.

Falk, K., Swedberg, K., Gaston-Johansson, F., *et al.* (2006) Fatigue and anaemia in patients with chronic heart failure. *European Journal of Heart Failure*, 8, 744–9.

Faris, R., Flather, M., Purcell, H., *et al.* (2002) Current evidence supporting the role of diuretics in heart failure: a meta-analysis of randomised controlled trials. *International Journal of Cardiology*, 82, 149–58.

Flather, M.D., Yusuf, S., Lober, L., *et al.* (ACE-Inhibitor Myocardial Infarction Collaborative Group) (2000) Long-term ACE-inhibitor therapy in patients with heart failure or left ventricular dysfunction: a systematic overview of data from individual patients. *Lancet*, 355(9215), 1575–81.

Gademan, M.G.J., Swenne, C.A., Verwey, H.F., *et al.* (2007) Effect of exercise training on autonomic derangement and neurohumoral activation in chronic heart failure. *Journal of Cardiac Heart Failure*, 13, 294–303.

Goldberg, R.J., Ciampa, J., Lessard, D., *et al.* (2007) Long term survival after heart failure. *Archives of Internal Medicine*, 167, 490–96.

Graves, J.E., Franklin, B. (eds) (2001) *Resistance Training for Health and Rehabilitation.* Champaign, IL: Human Kinetics.

Guazzi, M., Areana, R., Ascione, A., *et al.* (2007) Exercise oscillatory breathing and increased ventilation to carbon dioxide production slope in heart failure. *American Heart Journal,* 153, 859–67.

Guyatt, G.H. (1993) Measurement of health-related quality of life in heart failure. *Journal of the American College of Cardiology,* 22, 185a–91a.

Guyatt, G.H., Pugsley, S.O., Sullivan, M.J., *et al.* (1984) Effect of encouragement on walking test performance. *Thorax,* 39, 818–22.

Hambrecht, R., Gielen, S., Linke, A., *et al.* (2000) Effects of exercise training on left ventricular function and peripheral resistance in patients with chronic heart failure. *Journal of the American Medical Association,* 283, 3095–101.

Harrington, D., Anker, S.D., Chua, T.P. (1997). Skeletal muscle function and its relation to exercise tolerance in chronic heart failure. *Journal of the American College of Cardiology,* 30, 1758–64.

Haykowsky, M.J., Liang, Y., Pechter, D., *et al.* (2007) A meta-analysis of the effect of exercise training on left ventricular remodelling in heart failure patients. *Journal of the American College of Cardiology,* 49, 2329–36.

Hunt, S.A., Abraham, W.T., Chin, M.H., *et al.* (2005) ACC/AHA guideline update for the diagnosis and management of chronic heart failure in the adult: a report of the American College of Cardiology/American Heart Association. *Circulation,* 112, 1825–52.

Hunt, S.M., McKenna, S.P., McEwen, J., *et al.* (1980) A quantitative approach to perceived health status: a validation study. *Journal of Epidemiological Community Health,* 34, 281–6.

Ingle, L. (2007) Theoretical rationale and practical recommendations for cardiopulmonary exercise testing in patients with chronic heart failure. *Heart Failure Reviews,* 12, 12–22.

Ingle, L., Rigby, A.S., Carroll, S., *et al.* (2007) Prognostic value of the 6 minute walk tests and self-perceived symptom severity in older patients with chronic heart failure. *European Heart Journal,* 28, 560–68.

Jackson, G., Gibbs, C.R., Davies, M.K., *et al.* (2000) ABC of heart failure: pathophysiology. *British Medical Journal,* 320, 167–70.

Javaheri, S., Shukla, R., Zeigler, H., *et al.* (2007) Central sleep apnea, right ventricular dysfunction, and low diastolic blood pressure are predictors of mortality in systolic heart failure. *Journal of the American College of Cardiology,* 49, 2028–34.

Johansson, P., Agnebrink, M., Dahlström, U., *et al.* (2004) Measurement of health-related quality of life in chronic heart failure from a nursing perspective – a review of the literature. *European Journal of Cardiovascular Nursing,* 3, 7–20.

Johnson, P.H., Cowley, A.J., Kinnear, W.J. (1998) A randomized controlled trial of inspiratory muscle training in stable chronic heart failure. *European Heart Journal,* 19, 1249–53.

Kamalesh, M. (2006) Decreased survival in diabetic patients with heart failure due to systolic dysfunction. *European Journal of Heart Failure,* 8, 404–8.

Konstantinos, A.V., Tokmakidis, S.P. (2005) Resistance exercise training in patients with heart failure. *Sports Medicine,* 35, 1085–103.

Lang, C.C., Mancini, D.M. (2007) Non-cardiac co-morbidities in chronic heart failure. *Heart,* 93, 665–71.

Lloyd-Jones, D.M., Larson, M.G., Leip, E.P., *et al.* (2002) Lifetime risk for developing congestive heart failure: the Framingham heart study. *Circulation*, 106, 3068–72.

Mancini, D.M., Walter, G., Reichek, N. (1992) Contribution of skeletal muscle atrophy to exercise tolerance and altered muscle metabolism in heart failure. *Circulation*, 85, 1364–73.

Martos, R. (2007) Diastolic heart failure: evidence of increased myocardial collagen turnover linked to diastolic dysfunction. *Circulation*, 115, 888–95.

Mathew, P. (1998) Physical training in patients with ventricular dysfunction: choice and dosage of physical exercise in patients with pump dysfunction. *European Heart Journal*, 9 (Suppl F, 2), 67–9.

Mears, S. (2006) The importance of exercise training in patients with chronic heart failure. *Nursing Standard*, 20, 41–7.

Mettauer, B., Zoll, J., Garnier, A., *et al.* (2006) Heart failure: a model of cardiac and skeletal muscle energetic failure. Pflugers Archive. *European Journal of Physiology*, 452, 653–6.

Meyer, K., Bŭcking, J. (2004) Exercise in heart failure: should aqua therapy and swimming be allowed? *Medicine and Science in Sports and Exercise*, 36, 2017–23.

Meyer, K., Görnandt, L., Schwaibold, M., *et al.* (1997a) Predictors of response to exercise training in severe chronic congestive heart failure. *American Journal of Cardiology*, 80, 56–60.

Meyer, K., Samek, L., Schwaibold, M., *et al.* (1997b) Physical responses to different modes of interval exercise in patients with chronic heart failure – application to exercise training. *European Heart Journal*, 17, 1040–47.

Meyer, K., Schwaibold, M., Westbrook, S., *et al.* (1996) Effects of short-term exercise training and activity restriction on functional capacity in patients with severe chronic congestive heart failure. *American Journal of Cardiology*, 78, 1017–22.

Meyer, T., Kindermann, M., Kindermann, W. (2004) Exercise programmes for patients with chronic heart failure. *Sports Medicine*, 34, 939–54.

Mitchell, J.E. (2007) Emerging role of anaemia in heart failure. *American Journal of Cardiology*, 99 (Suppl), 15D–20D.

Moser, D.K., Worster, P.L. (2000) Effect of psychosocial factors on physiologic outcomes in patients with heart failure. *Journal of Cardiovascular Nursing*, 14, 106–15.

Myers, J. (2008) Principles of exercise prescription for patients with chronic heart failure. *Heart Failure Reviews*, 13(1), 61–8.

Myers, J., Hadley, D., Oswald, U., *et al.* (2007) Effects of exercise training on heart rate recovery in patients with chronic heart failure. *American Heart Journal*, 153, 1056–63.

National Institute of Clinical Excellence (NICE) (2003) *Chronic Heart Failure – National Clinical Guideline for Diagnosis and Management in Primary and Secondary Care*. Guideline No. 5. London: Royal College of Physicians.

Nichols, G. (2001) Congestive heart failure in type 2 diabetes: prevalence, incidence, and risk factors. *Diabetes Care*, 24, 1614–19.

Nolan, J., Batin, P.D., Andrews, R., *et al.* (1998) Prospective study of heart rate variability and mortality in chronic heart failure: Results of the United Kingdom heart failure evaluation and assessment of risk trial (UK-heart). *Circulation*, 98(15), 1510–16.

Oka, R.K., Stotts, N.A., Dae, M.W., *et al.* (1993) Daily physical activity levels in congestive heart failure. *American Journal of Cardiology*, 71, 921–5.

Oldenburg, O., Lamp, B., Faber, L., *et al.* (2007) Sleep-disordered breathing in patients with symptomatic heart failure. *European Journal of Heart Failure*, 9, 251–7.

Olson, T.P., Synder, E.M., Johnson, B.D. (2006) Exercise-disordered breathing in chronic heart failure. *Exercise and Sport Sciences Reviews*, 34, 194–201.

Passantino, A., Lagioia, R., Mastropasqua, F., *et al.* (2006) Short-term change in distance walked in 6 minute is an indicator of outcome in patients with chronic heart failure in clinical practice. *Journal of the American College of Cardiology*, 48, 99–105.

Physiotools (2005) *Cardiovascular and Flexibility Exercise.* Finland. Available from http://www.toolsrg.com.

Piepoli, M., Coats, A.J. (1996) Autonomic abnormality in chronic heart failure evaluated by heart rate variability. *Clinical Science*, 91 (Suppl), 84–6.

Piepoli, M., Kaczmarek, A., Francis, D.P., *et al.* (2006) Reduced peripheral skeletal muscle mass and abnormal reflex physiology in chronic heart failure. *Circulation*, 114, 126–34.

Piña, I.L., Apstein, C.S., Balady, G.J., *et al.* (2003) Exercise and heart failure: a statement from the American Heart Association committee on exercise, rehabilitation and prevention. *Circulation*, 107, 1210–25.

Poole-Wilson, P.A., Buller, N.P., Lindsay, D.C. (1992) Blood flow and skeletal muscle in patients with heart failure. *Chest*, 101 (Suppl), 330S–32S.

Quinones, M.A., Zile, M.R., Massie, B.M., *et al.* (For the Participants of the Dartmouth Diastole Discourses) (2006) Chronic heart failure: a report from Participants of the Dartmouth Diastole Discourses. *Congestive Heart Failure*, 12, 162–5.

Rector, T.S., Kubo, S.H., Cohn, J.N. (1987) Patient's self assessment of their congestive heart failure: content, reliability, and validity of a new measure: the Minnesota Living with Heart Failure questionnaire. *Heart Failure*, 3, 198–219.

Rees, K., Taylor, R.S., Singh, S., *et al.* (2004) Exercise based rehabilitation for heart failure. *Cochrane Database Systematic Reviews*, 3, CD003331.

Remme, W.J., Swedberg, K. (2001) Guidelines for the diagnosis and treatment of chronic heart failure. *European Heart Journal*, 22, 1527–60.

Schaulfelberger, M., Eriksson, B.O., Grimby, G. (1997) Skeletal muscle alterations in patients with chronic heart failure. *European Heart Journal*, 18, 971–80.

Scottish Intercollegiate Guidelines Network (SIGN) (2002) *Cardiac Rehabilitation – A National Clinical Guideline, No. 57.* Edinburgh, UK: SIGN.

Scottish Intercollegiate Guidelines Network (SIGN) (2007a) *Management of Chronic Heart Failure – A National Clinical Guideline, No. 95.* Edinburgh, UK: SIGN.

Scottish Intercollegiate Guidelines Network (SIGN) (2007b) *Risk Estimation and the Prevention of Cardiovascular Disease – A National Clinical Guideline, No. 97.* Edinburgh, UK: SIGN.

Singh, S.J., Morgan, M.D.L., Scott, S., *et al.* (1992) Development of a shuttle walking test of disability in patients with chronic airways obstruction. *Thorax*, 47, 1019–24.

Smart, N.A., Fang, Z.Y., Marwick, T.H. (2003) A practical guide to exercise training for heart failure patients. *Journal of Cardiac Failure*, 9, 49–58.

Smart, N.A., Marwick, T.H. (2004) Exercise training for heart failure patients: a systematic review of factors that improve mortality and morbidity. *American Journal of Medicine*, 116, 693–706.

Solway, S., Brooks, D., Lacasse, Y., *et al.* (2001) Qualitative systematic overview of the measurement properties of functional walking tests used in the cardiorespiratory domain. *Chest*, 119, 256–70.

Specchia, G., DeServi, S., Scire, A., *et al.* (1996) Coronary heart disease/ atherosclerosis/myocardial infarction: interaction between exercise training and ejection fraction in predicting prognosis after first myocardial infarction. *Circulation*, 94, 978–82.

Stassijns, G. (1996) Peripheral and respiratory muscles in chronic heart failure. *European Respiration Journal*, 9, 2161–7.

Stewart, K.J., Badenhop D., Brubaker, P.H., *et al.* (2003) Cardiac rehabilitation following percutaneous revascularisation, heart transplant, heart valve surgery, and for chronic heart failure. *Chest*, 123, 2104–11.

Taylor, A. (1999) Physiological response to a short period of exercise training in patients with chronic heart failure. *Physiotherapy Research International*, 4, 237–49.

Thow, M.K. (ed.) (2006) *Exercise Leadership in Cardiac Rehabilitation – An Evidence-Based Approach.* West Sussex: Wiley and Sons.

Tobin, D., Thow, M.K. (1999) The 10 m shuttle walk test with holter monitoring: an objective outcome measure for cardiac rehabilitation. *Coronary Health Care*, 3, 3–17.

Torchio, R., Gulotta, C., Greco-Lucchina, P., *et al.* (2006) Closing capacity and gas exchange in chronic heart failure. *Chest*, 129, 1330–36.

Van Den Berg-Emons, R., Bussmann, J., Balk, A., *et al.* (2001) Level of activities associated with mobility during everyday life in patients with chronic congestive heart failure as measured with an 'Activity Monitor'. *Physical Therapy*, 81, 1502–11.

Van Den Berg-Emons, R., Balk, A., Bussman, H., *et al.* (2004) Does aerobic training lead to a more active lifestyle and improved quality of life in patients with chronic heart failure? *European Journal of Heart Failure*, 6, 95–100.

Van Den Berg-Emons, R., Bussmann, J., Balk, A., *et al.* (2005) Factors associated with the level of movement-related everyday activity and quality of life in people with chronic heart failure. *Physical Therapy*, 85, 1340–48.

Van Der Ent, M., Jeneson, J.A.L, Remme, W.J. (1998) A non-invasive selective assessment of type I fibre mitochondrial function using ^{31}P NMR spectroscopy: evidence for impaired oxidative phosphorylation rate in skeletal muscle in patients with chronic heart failure. *European Heart Journal*, 19, 124–31.

Velloso, M., Jardim, J.R. (2006) Functionality of patients with chronic obstructive pulmonary disease: energy conservation techniques. *Jornal Brasileiro De Pneumologia*, 32, 580–86.

Vescovo, G., Dalla Libera, L. (2006). Skeletal muscle apoptosis in experimental heart failure: the only link between inflammation and skeletal muscle wastage? *Current Opinions in Clinical Nutrition Metabolic Care*, 9, 416–22.

Wang, H., Parker, J.D., Newton, G.E., *et al.* (2007) Influence of obstructive sleep apnea on mortality in patients with heart failure. *Journal of the American College of Cardiology*, 49, 1625–31.

Ware, J.E., Sherbourne, C.D. (1992) The MOS 36-item short-form health survey (SF 36): conceptual framework and item selection. *Medical Care*, 30, 473–85.

Weiner, P., Waizman, J., Magadle, R., *et al.* (1999) The effect of specific inspiratory muscle training on the sensation of dyspnea and exercise tolerance in patients with congestive heart failure. *Clinical Cardiology*, 22, 727–32.

Whellan, D.J., O'Connor, C.M., Lee, K.L., *et al.* (2007) Heart failure and a controlled trial investigating outcomes of exercise training (HF-ACTION): design and rationale. *American Heart Journal*, 153, 201–11.

Wisløff, U., Støylen, A., Loennechen, J.P., *et al.* (2007) Superior cardiovascular effect of aerobic interval training versus moderate continuous training in heart failure patients. *Circulation*, 225, 3086–94.

You Fang, Z. (2003) Mechanisms of exercise training in patients with heart failure. *American Heart Journal*, 145, 904–11.

Zile, M.R., LeWinter, M.M. (2007) Left ventricular end-diastolic volume is normal in patients with heart failure and a normal ejection fraction. *Journal of the American College of Cardiology*, 49, 982–5.

4 Arrhythmia and Implanted Cardioverter Defibrillators

Patrick Doherty and Samantha Breen

Chapter outline

This chapter reviews the pathophysiology of sudden cardiac death and arrhythmia. This is followed by evidence-based clinical guidance regarding the efficacy of physical activity and exercise in the management of patients with arrhythmia and specifically those fitted with an implantable cardioverter defibrillator (ICD). The relationship between physical activity and exercise and associated recommendations in secondary prevention and public health are discussed. Traditional misconceptions concerning exercise are challenged and evidence-based solutions offered. Guidelines on exercise programme design are presented and justified. The emphasis of the chapter is on developing safe, pragmatic and practical advice that clinicians and patients can use in decision-making about physical activity and exercise.

Pathophysiology and incidence of sudden cardiac death

Arrhythmia is an abnormality of the heart's rhythm that alters the normal electrical activity of the heart. The heart may beat slow, fast or just beat irregularly, and this can result in breathlessness, dizziness and/or loss of consciousness (DH, 2005). Cardiac arrest or sudden cardiac death (SCD) is less well known than heart attack and very different is its presentation. The National Institute for Clinical Excellence definition of SCD is as follows:

> An abrupt loss of consciousness and unexpected death due to cardiac causes, which occur within one hour of onset of symptoms (NICE, 2000, p. 2).

Tachyarrhythmias cause about 80% of SCD events in the form of ventricular tachycardia (VT) and ventricular fibrillation (VF), and these can be independent of reduced vascular flow or blockage and therefore contrast with the origins of heart attack or myocardial infarction (MI). Patients with arrhythmia are highly likely to suffer sudden death and are considered at high risk of such an event in any aspect of their day. Out of the 300 000 deaths attributed to coronary heart disease (CHD) each year in the UK, approximately 3 out of 10 are SCDs. The rate of SCD (cardiac arrest) is estimated at a maximum of 70 000–100 000 per year in the UK, with 80% of arrhythmias due to ventricular tachyarrhythmia, and heart failure is strongly associated with arrhythmia (Bryant et al., 2005; NICE, 2007). In Britain, survival is estimated at 5% if a hospital is reached and 2% for out-of-hospital SCD episodes. Survivors of SCD are likely to have a recurrence within 1 year, which is often fatal (NICE, 2007).

High-risk patients with arrhythmia or a strong likelihood of arrhythmias including those with heart failure can benefit from physical activity and exercise as part of cardiac rehabilitation (CR) (Fitchet et al., 2003; Lampman and Knight, 2000; Rees et al., 2004; Smart and Marwick, 2004; Vanhees et al., 2001). This chapter sets out to clarify some of the uncertainty that exists in regard to advising these patients about exercise.

Likelihood of arrhythmia during exercise

Exercise-induced arrhythmia continues to be a possibility in patients with arrhythmia at the start of exercise, during and at the end of exercise, and is influenced by decreased vagal tone, latency of the sympathetic nervous system, circulating catecholamines and excessive myocardial demand (Beckerman et al., 2005; Belardinelli, 2003; Braith and Edwards, 2003; Malfatto et al., 1996; Mayordomo and Batalla, 2002). The potential for exercise to induce arrhythmia increases if the person is a patient with a cardiac condition and suffering from anxiety. The psychological state of anxiety has a part to play during the initial and more intense levels of exercise. The mechanism is, however, unknown (Sears et al., 2001). The incidence of arrhythmia during intense exercise in well documented and is not purely pathological in origin (Fleg et al., 2000; MacAuley, 1999; Pashkow et al., 1997). The risk of both exercise-related MI and sudden death is greatest in individuals who are the least physically active and still performing unaccustomed vigorous physical activity. Exercise can induce or prevent arrhythmia, and exercise training lessens the likelihood of arrhythmia (Belardinelli, 2003; Malfatto et al., 1996). Regular moderate exercise over an 8-week period in post-MI patients has been shown to improve parasympathetic tone, increase heart rate (HR) variability, reduce the incidence of arrhythmia and improve prognosis (Malfatto et al., 1996). Cardiorespiratory fitness training and strength training can be performed safely and effectively in patients with arrhythmias (Fitchet et al., 2003; Vanhees et al., 2001). A summary of the factors contributing to the likelihood of arrhythmia during exercise and in turn influenced by exercise is shown in Figure 4.1. Although the literature offers a range of views on the benefits of exercise, what can be said is that moderate exercise is well tolerated and beneficial if performed routinely.

The likelihood of exercise provoking arrhythmia is greatest in patients with cardiac disease as the extremes of exercise are reached, especially

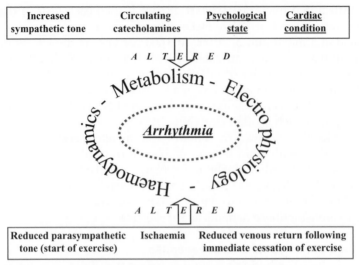

| Increased sympathetic tone | Circulating catecholamines | Psychological state | Cardiac condition |

A L T E R E D

Metabolism - Electrophysiology - Haemodynamics

Arrhythmia

A L T E R E D

| Reduced parasympathetic tone (start of exercise) | Ischaemia | Reduced venous return following immediate cessation of exercise |

Figure 4.1 Factors that influence the likelihood of arrhythmia during exercise.

in patients who are novices to the mode of exercise. Figure 4.2 and Table 4.1 show the exercise test outcome for all patients referred for treadmill exercise testing and suggest that on average approximately 4.2% of patients are likely to present with arrhythmia during high levels of exertion (mean of 8.7 METs). This intensity relates to sustaining a walking intensity of 3.4 miles/hour on a 14% gradient, which is a challenge for most people over the age of 50 years. Box 4.1 summarises risk in respect of exercise and key messages to reduce risk during exercise.

Performance of patients with arrhythmia during exercise

Exercise professionals in CR are often concerned about exercising a patient with known arrhythmia because the consequence of poorly performed exercise at a relatively high intensity could be a cardiac arrest, which in most cases is fatal. The important point, in terms of CR, is that clinicians are often exercising patients well below the intensities associated with exercise-induced arrhythmias. Table 4.2 shows that patients with a history of arrhythmia, primarily involving the ventricles, on average, perform well during exercise. A history of breathlessness or unmanaged acute atrial fibrillation is far more limiting in terms of exercise capacity. In approximately 28% of patients with known arrhythmia, exercise testing is provocative and leads to arrhythmia either during or immediately following exercise. The average MET associated with arrhythmia in this at-risk subgroup of patients was 9.4 (SD 2.5). Using the physical activity compendium, this would enable most of these patients to run a 12-min/mile (Ainsworth *et al.*, 1993). CR exercise, even performed at its highest levels, is less intensive

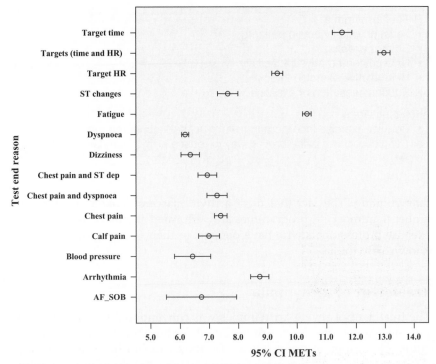

Figure 4.2 Treadmill exercise test outcomes, in metabolic equivalents (METs), for 5445 referred cardiac patients (mean age of 54 years) (Manchester Heart Centre Data, 2007).

Table 4.1 Treadmill exercise outcome, in metabolic equivalents (METs), for referred cardiac patients (mean age of 54 years).

Test end reason	Mean	SD	N	% of total N
AF_SOB	6.7	2.6	20	0.4
Arrhythmia	8.7	2.4	229	4.2
Blood pressure	6.4	2.1	46	0.8
Calf pain	7.0	2.3	158	2.9
Chest pain	7.4	2.3	438	8.0
Chest pain and dyspnoea	7.3	2.4	183	3.4
Chest pain and ST depression	6.9	2.0	147	2.7
Dizziness	6.4	2.1	163	3.0
Fatigue	10.3	3.0	1687	31.0
Dyspnoea	6.2	1.7	751	13.8
ST changes	7.6	2.3	175	3.2
Target HR	9.3	2.7	784	14.4
Target time	11.5	2.4	205	3.8
Targets (time and HR)	13.0	2.3	459	8.4
Total	9.0	3.2	5445	100.0

Manchester Heart Centre data (2007).

Box 4.1 Risk of arrhythmia and key messages.

Risk of arrhythmia
- Least physically active patients
- Start of exercise
- Unaccustomed physical activity
- High relative exercise intensity
- Sudden cessation of exercise

Key messages
- Regular exercise incorporating warm-up, self-monitored moderate intensity and cool-down is the proven way to reduce arrhythmia risk during exercise

than running. The fact that most arrhythmias are evoked at intensities higher than most CR programmes are performed should be reassuring to exercise professionals who have patients in their CR programme with a known arrhythmia.

Treatment of arrhythmia

The treatment of severe arrhythmias was conventionally by antiarrhythmic medication and the use of hospital-based cardioversion as required. Although a range of drugs is used for the treatment of arrhythmia, evidence suggests that conventional treatment would include antiarrhythmic medication, most commonly amiodarone and β-blockade. Treatment by medication is less effective than ICDs at reducing arrhythmic death (Parkes *et al.*, 2000). However, neither treatment approach, either in isolation or in

Table 4.2 Exercise test outcome where the test reason is ventricular arrhythmia.

Test end reason	Mean	SD	N	% of total N
Arrhythmia	9.4	2.5	78	27.6
Calf pain	4.0		1	0.4
Chest pain	4.6	0.6	2	0.7
Chest pain and dyspnoea	5.4	2.1	4	1.4
Dizziness	8.4	3.7	6	2.1
Fatigue	12.6	3.3	83	29.3
Dyspnoea	6.4	1.6	13	4.6
ST changes	7.5	4.1	2	0.7
Target HR	10.8	3.4	45	15.9
Target time	14.0	2.3	6	2.1
Targets (time and HR)	13.5	2.2	43	15.2
Total	11.0	3.6	283	100.0

Manchester Heart Centre data (2007).

combination, can reduce mortality to the extent that these patients feel safe with exercise or moderate physical activity (Sears *et al.*, 2001). Poor heart function accompanies severe acute or chronic arrhythmia and is often reflected in a reduced left ventricular ejection fraction (LVEF) of less than 35%. Such low output from the ventricles (70–80% being normal) and associated poor haemodynamics leads to considerable deficit in functional capacity or ability to perform physical work (Coats *et al.*, 1992; Fleg *et al.*, 2000; Gibbons *et al.*, 2002; NICE, 2000).

The evidence points to a 50% reduction in arrhythmic death with the use of an ICD in cardiac arrest survivors and patients with low ejection fraction following MI (Bryant *et al.*, 2005).

Evidence for the effectiveness of ICDs is clear in the secondary prevention of SCD, and strong evidence is now developing for their primary role in SCD. This is echoed in the recommendations from NICE and the Department of Health for a substantial increase in the number of ICDs to be fitted in the next few years (DH, 2005; NICE, 2000). Both these guidelines acknowledge that exercise and rehabilitation are presently not offered post-implantation and recommend that implanting centres should now offer and evaluate a rehabilitative approach.

During the development of the new arrhythmia chapter for DH (2005) NSF, it became clear that patients and exercise professionals were concerned about the lack of information regarding exercise and physical activity (DH, 2005). Patients were, in many situations, advised initially to do very little physical activity and to increase activity gradually, the caveat being to stop if they encountered any difficulties (Sears *et al.*, 1999, 2001). Clinically, it is apparent that the passage of time since implant does not resolve the psychosocial issues and fear of ICD shocks during exercise and physical activity. Over half the patients presently fitted with an ICD will have had the device implanted for over 5 years, which represents a substantial period of inactivity. Equally, there appears to be a rapid loss in functional capacity in some patients, and a general sedentary status continues to be a major concern.

Implantable cardioverter defibrillators

The history of ICDs is relatively short, as Dr Michel Mirowski first considered them in 1969, when external defibrillators were becoming the modality of choice for the treatment of arrhythmia and cardiac arrest (SCD episode) in coronary care units. The use of implanted pacemakers was relatively common, and it seemed logical to Mirowski, although not to most of his peers, that it would be feasible and safe to miniaturise the defibrillator (Singer, 1994). Dr Mirowski and Dr Morton Mower combined forces from 1972 to 1980 at the Sinai Hospital in Baltimore to develop and implant the first defibrillator in a dog in 1976. The pictures of a dog collapsed due to syncope via an induced arrhythmia and then on its feet within seconds of

Table 4.3 New York Heart Association functional classification.

Class	Description
I	No limitation of activity; ordinary activity does not cause symptoms
II	Slight limitation of activity; ordinary activity results in symptoms
II	Marked limitation of activity; less than ordinary activity results in symptoms
IV	Unable to carry on any physical activity without discomfort; symptoms at rest

Fletcher *et al.* (2001).

the automated defibrillator firing are impressive even now. Approval was soon given to implant the first ICD in a human being, and the procedure was first successfully performed in February 1980.

ICD implantation criteria

The two most important ICD patient implantation selection criteria alongside arrhythmia were LVEF and the New York Heart Association (NYHA) Functional Classification (Table 4.3). LVEF represents the amount of blood (percentage of total ventricular volume) ejected from the ventricle during systole. A healthy heart would eject in the region of 70–80% of its ventricular blood volume, whereas a patient with an LVEF of less than 35% would be considered severely compromised (Coats *et al.*, 1992; Singer, 1994). The NYHA classification was originally derived and validated from interviewing heart failure patients regarding the limitation of activity and the presentation of symptoms (e.g. dyspnoea) during their day.

The NYHA system is simple and inexpensive and has demonstrated substantial predictive validity (Fletcher *et al.*, 2001; Gibbons *et al.*, 2002).

The use of the NYHA functional classification within chronic arrhythmia and heart failure patients has increased, as more patients are being considered for ICDs as part of primary prevention of SCD. Although the NYHA functional class has been criticised for its subjective nature and imprecision when distinguishing between class II and class III (Fleg *et al.*, 2000), the system is well used and easily understood (Gibbons *et al.*, 1997). The subjectivity of the NYHA functional class is less of a concern when acting alongside LVEF as one of the criteria for ICD implantation, as this should counterbalance any discrepancies within the NYHA rating (DH, 2005; NICE, 2000). Currently in the UK the criteria for ICD implantation are set out by the NICE (2007) as shown in Table 4.4.

Evidence for the benefit of ICDs

The effectiveness of ICDs has been proved through randomised controlled trials, and the following section elaborates the salient points, with a summary at the end of the section (Table 4.5).

Table 4.4 ICD implantation criteria.

NICE secondary prevention ICD implantation criteria	NICE primary prevention ICD implantation criteria

1. Cardiac arrest due to VT or VF
 	
2. Spontaneous sustained VT associated with syncope and haemodynamic compromise
 	
3. Sustained VT without syncope/compromise with EF <35%, NYHA III/IV
	1. History of previous (>4 weeks) MI and either
	    LV dysfunction <35% and non-sustained VT on Holter monitoring and inducible VT on EP testing
	or
	    LV dysfunction with LVEF <30% and QRS duration equal to or more than 120 milliseconds
	
	2. Familial condition with high risk of sudden death: long QT syndrome, hypertrophic cardiomyopathy, Brugada syndrome and arrhythmogenic RV dysplasia

NICE (2007).

Table 4.5 Summary of defibrillator trials.

Trial	Start date	Comparison	N	Primary outcome: total mortality
CASH	1987	ICD vs CT	400	37% reduction at 2 years compared with CT
CIDS	1990	ICD vs amiodarone	184	Non-published
MADIT	1991	ICD vs CT	95 and 101	ICD 54% reduction
AVID	1993	ICD vs CT	1016	ICD 39% reduction year 1 ICD 27% reduction year 2 ICD 31% reduction year 3
MUSTT	1993	EPs (ICD vs CT) vs NT	704	ICD 51% reduction in all-cause mortality vs NT. CT vs NT no change
DEBUT	1997	β-blockade vs ICD	61	14% increase for β-blockade, 0% mortality ICD
MADIT II	1998	ICD vs no ICD Post-MI, LVEF <30%	1232	30% reduction in mortality (20 months mean follow-up)
BEST-ICD	1999	CT vs EPs with (CT vs ICD) split	1200	Non-published
CABG patch	1996	CABG vs ICDs plus CABG	900	No evidence of prophylaxis

CT, conventional treatment (β-blockade plus amiodarone); EPs, electrophysiological studies; NT, no treatment.

The Cardiac Arrest Study Hamburg (CASH) investigated antiarrhythmic drugs versus ICDs. The study had three comparative drugs within the antiarrhythmic aspect: metoprolol, amiodarone and propafenone (Siebels and Kuck, 1994). The propafenone drug in this study was stopped due to significant mortality compared to the ICD aspect of the study, and the study continued with the other comparisons. The 2-year preliminary findings found ICDs to have a 37% reduction in mortality compared to the remaining antiarrhythmic groups.

The Canadian Implantable Defibrillator Study (CIDS) compared ICDs with amiodarone. A total of 659 patients who survived cardiac arrest due to VF or VT or with unmonitored syncope were randomly assigned to treatment with the ICD or with amiodarone. The study concluded that ICD therapy conferred a 20% relative risk reduction in all-cause mortality and a 33% reduction in arrhythmic mortality when compared to amiodarone (Connolly *et al.*, 2000).

The Multicenter Autonomic Defibrillator Trial (MADIT) considered the primary prophylactic role of ICDs against combinations of antiarrhythmic therapy in 196 high-risk patients. Selection criteria were the NYHA functional class I, II, or III, unsustained VT, previous MI and an LVEF ≤35%. Baseline characteristics were similar between groups and on average they were followed up for 27 months. There were 15 deaths in the ICD group (11 from cardiac causes) and 39 deaths (27 from cardiac causes) in the conventional therapy groups. In post-MI patients with a high risk for ventricular tachyarrhythmias, prophylactic therapy with an implanted defibrillator was associated with improved survival compared with conventional medical therapy. Antiarrhythmic drug therapy had no influence on the mortality and ICDs reduced mortality by 54%. These findings led to a financial appraisal of the prophylactic use of ICDs, which concluded that the evidence was insufficient to warrant investment.

Multicenter Autonomic Defibrillator Trial II (MADIT II) considered high-risk CHD patients with low LVEF (<30%) and an NYHA rating between class I and class III. Patients were all on optimal drug therapy. Reduced LVEF overcame some of the concerns expressed by Moss *et al.* (1996), where the greatest benefit and most appropriate selection was associated with low ejection fraction. The study evaluated the primary preventative role of ICDs in reducing SCD and involved a defibrillator group of 742 patients (84% male), mean age of 64 (SD 10), and a conventional therapy group of 490 patients (85% male), mean age of 65 (SD 10). Although planned as a 5-year trial, the study terminated at 4 years (20 months mean follow-up) due to a 30% reduction in mortality for post-MI patients receiving an ICD compared to those receiving conventional treatment. The study concluded that ICDs in this class of patient have a strong prophylactic role and should be considered as a recommended therapy (Myers *et al.*, 2007).

One of the largest initial studies was the antiarrhythmic versus implantable defibrillator (AVID). AVID was powered for a sample size of 2500, yet the trial was terminated early with a sample of 1016 due to a significant reduction in mortality for the ICD group. The authors extrapolated their findings and estimated that 1000 lives would be saved per year in high-risk patients with the use of ICDs. There were 122 and 80 deaths in the antiarrhythmic drugs and ICD conditions, respectively. This represents an overall arrhythmic death of 39%, irrespective of optimal antiarrhythmic drugs or an ICD, and highlights that ICDs are not a guarantee of survival. Hallstrom *et al.* (2001) reanalysed the AVID data in relation to the baseline characteristics and found greater benefit for patients with a prior history of arrhythmia and low LVEF (<35%).

The primary use of ICDs to prevent SCD was the focus of the Coronary Artery Bypass Graft Patch (CABG Patch) trial. The patch refers to the location of the ICD within the epicardial region. ICDs were randomly implanted into 446 of 900 patients undergoing CABG. Within 32 months the study was terminated, as there was no evidence for the prophylactic use of ICDs (Curtis *et al.*, 1997). There is some debate regarding the definition of high risk in the CABG Patch trial compared to MADIT, with ejection fraction criteria being 36 and 35%, respectively. Notwithstanding this, the study was the first negative finding.

The Beta-Blockade Strategy plus Implantable Cardioverter Defibrillator (BEST-ICD) Trial, although presently recruiting, plans to evaluate the use of electrophysiological studies (EPs) to guide prescription towards optimal β-blockade and ICD therapy. With the exception of MUSTT, previous trials have not considered the possible effect that EPs were having on the outcome, as EPs were only applied to the ICD patients. The permutations and subset sample size of BEST-ICD are more appropriate for answering this question than MUSTT (Raviele *et al.*, 1999). Table 4.5 summarises defibrillator studies.

Parkes *et al.* (2000) performed a systematic review of ICD efficacy as part of a health technology assessment of the NICE (2000) guidance. They initially reviewed 1610 abstracts and reduced this to 17 papers where the data were extracted for the analysis. Collectively, ICDs can reduce mortality considerably. However, there is a confidence interval ranging between 1.7 and 22.8%.

The best outcome, in terms of decreased mortality, appears to occur in patients with low LVEF, hypertrophic cardiomyopathy and familial arrhythmias such as Brugada syndrome. The study concluded that on average the ICD secondary role towards reducing SCD was well supported, with a primary role indicated.

An important point to take from these trials is that patients will still die prematurely with an ICD fitted, and it is important not to see the device as a guaranteed lifesaver. Good advice on, and facilitation of, health-related physical activity and exercise will, in the long-term, save more lives than an ICD.

Defibrillator implantation

Early devices were fitted by surgeons using classical thoracic access routes. However, these have been replaced by less dramatic methods, using approaches developed from the clinical experience with electrocardio-physiological techniques. Miniaturisation of ICDs and transvenous entry have lessened the aftercare required. ICDs tend to be fitted beneath (inferior to) the clavicle, either under the pectoris major in a fascial pouch or above the muscle and beneath the adipose fascia of the dermis (Figure 4.3, mode 1). Surgery is performed under local anaesthetic with a length of hospital stay between 1 and 3 days post-surgery, depending on the extent of ICD programming post-implant.

The device has a battery life in the newer models that ranges from 5 to 9 years, and replacement does not require the removal of the leads from the ventricles. Battery life is variable and can be prolonged by capacitor programming under the guidance of the ICD technician. Older devices continue to be replaced with newer models that are up to a third of the size, at 30–40 cm^3, weighing approximately 80 g and smaller than traditional pacemakers.

There is a second wave of ICDs being implanted subcutaneously to overcome some of the issues with infection in the veins that arise from the myocardial transvenous route. These devices are a basic 'shock box'

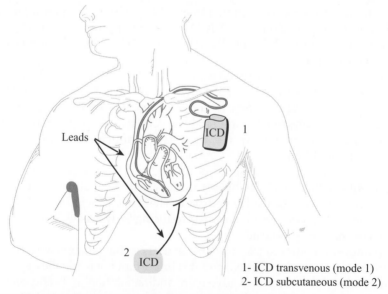

1- ICD transvenous (mode 1)
2- ICD subcutaneous (mode 2)

Figure 4.3 Implantable cardioverter defibrillator and implantation location.

that will simply deliver defibrillation to the myocardium via a single lead attached externally or through the viscera tissues via a transmission electrode (Figure 4.2, mode 2).

Types of ICD
The original ICD was designed to detect VF and deliver a high-energy shock (defibrillation) only, via a single lead implanted in the right ventricle. Advancements in technology in the early 1990s have introduced tiered therapies, where antitachycardia pacing and low-energy shocks (cardioversion) can be delivered for VT. There are three types of ICDs:
1. *Single-chamber ICD*: This device has a single lead attached in the right ventricle. Of these devices most can distinguish between sudden-onset sinus tachycardia and VT and can identify stability of the cardiac cycle lengths to detect atrial fibrillation. However, atrial arrhythmias may be responsible for approximately 50% of inappropriate shocks, which are less likely to be detected without an atrial lead (i.e. dual chamber).
2. *Dual-chamber ICD*: Dual-chamber devices were developed in the late 1990s. These devices have two leads: one attached in the right atrium and one in the right ventricle. The addition of an atrial lead enables atrial rhythm information to be used in the algorithm analysis, enabling enhanced diagnostics and resulting in reduced inappropriate shock therapy. These devices can deliver the following therapies:
   • Atrial tachycardia and atrial fibrillation detection
   • Bradycardia sensing and pacing
   • Antitachycardia pacing
   • Cardioversion
   • Defibrillation
3. *Biventricular ICD*: In 2000, cardiac resynchronisation therapy (CRT) was developed using biventricular pacing to improve heart function (Abraham *et al.*, 2002). Leads are attached as for the dual-chamber device, with an additional lead implanted onto the epicardial surface of the left ventricle. Therapy capabilities for the biventricular device are as for the dual-chamber with the addition of CRT. CRT has been shown to improve haemodynamic function, increase exercise tolerance and lower NYHA status in patients with a poor LVEF, intraventricular conduction delay and advanced heart failure (NYHA classes III and IV). Figure 4.3 shows the location of ICD and implantation.

As the ICD battery approaches its end point, the unit, with the exception of the wires, is replaced in a relatively minor procedure performed under local anaesthesia with mild sedation. Patients rarely require more than 1 day in hospital for a battery change procedure.

Incidence of ICD implantation
In 2000, the number of implants was 194 per million in the US, 17 per million in the UK and 13 per million in France (Figure 4.4). The NICE

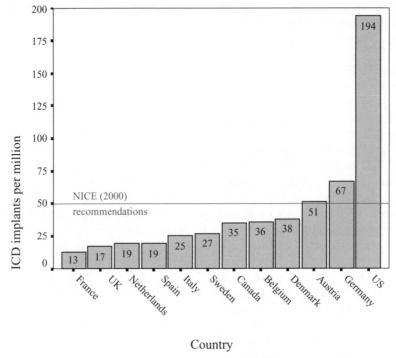

Figure 4.4 Implantation rates based on NICE (2000) recommendation.

guidelines recommend an increase from 17 to 50 per million in the UK, with an estimated cost of £49 million per year (NICE, 2007). This value, based on a £12 000 per device, assumes a total cost of £20 000, inclusive of associated services and overheads. These associated costs do not include CR, even though the NICE guidelines suggest that they include rehabilitation. The rate of ICD implantation is presently 43 per million (NICE, 2007) and is expected to increase further over the next 5 years. Clinicians are more likely than ever before to have patients with an ICD referred to their service.

Detection of arrhythmia and subsequent therapy

ICDs have two primary functions: firstly, to monitor rhythm via the sensing leads that carry signals back from the heart, and secondly, to deliver either mild antitachycardia pacing (ATP) or shock in response to life-threatening arrhythmias. The detection of arrhythmia, although related to the number of beats per minute, is based on milliseconds, with a resting HR of 60 beats/min equivalent to 1000 milliseconds. This represents a large discriminative range and enables a high degree of surveillance that requires advance computation and algorithms to detect and treat arrhythmia (Singer, 1994; Wilkoff, 2006).

ICDs deliver electrical energy to the heart at a high frequency that gradually dominates the rhythm and brings the rate down to a normal range, enabling sinoatrial node to take control again. The ICD can be programmed to react in four different ways to restore the heart rate and rhythm:

• *Antitachycardia pacing*: A series of small, rapid electrical pacing pulses or bursts delivered over shorter duration (milliseconds) interrupt the arrhythmia and return heart to its normal rhythm.

• *Cardioversion*: If the arrhythmia is regular but very fast, the ICD can deliver a low-energy shock. This interrupts the arrhythmia and returns the heart to its normal rhythm.

• *Defibrillation*: Arrhythmias that are very fast and irregular require high-energy shocks (range from 29 to 42 J) to stop the arrhythmia.

• *Pacemaker*: Dual-chamber rate-modulated pacing (DDD) or single-chamber rate-modulated ventricular pacing (VVVI) for bradyarrhythmias which are common post-shock.

The system monitors heart rate activity and activates the pulse generator when appropriate therapy is required. The issue of oversensing and inappropriate therapy is evident in the literature, with dual-chamber ICDs being considered more vigilant and arguably more responsive (Exner *et al.*, 2001; Pinski and Fahy, 1995; Wilkoff, 2006). The schematic in Figure 4.5 shows the combined options of many of the ICD programming strategies, with the platform being the monitor and standby mode.

For each ICD, the parameters are set specifically for each patient, dependent on the findings of the EPs (see Table 4.5 for example of defibrillator studies). The following represents the different types of rhythms being detected:

• VT   150–214 beats/min
• Fast VT   188–250 beats/min

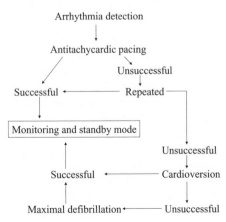

Figure 4.5 Schematic of ICD programming options.

- VF   188–500 beats/min
- DDD pacing   <40 beats/min

(VT, ventricular tachycardia; VF, ventricular fibrillation; DDD, dual-chamber rate-modulated pacing)

Interrogation of the ICD

A specialist ICD technician has the skills and software to interrogate the device by placing a pad connected to a computer over the chest wall, which can communicate with the ICD. The software holds millisecond history, which enables the technician to check for arrhythmias and ICD activity (ATP and shocks). Most importantly, it allows the technician to determine whether the therapy delivered by the ICD has been appropriate or not. Changes in medication or device therapy settings can be made on the basis of the information gleaned. The battery is also checked at each visit to ascertain how much energy remains. For devices that deliver a lot of therapy, the battery life will be shorter. Patients will have regular check-ups following device implantation and after any therapy that the device has delivered.

Inappropriate therapy

Inappropriate therapy is a real concern for some patients and for clinicians and exercise professionals. The anxiety relates to the association between repeated therapies delivered by ICDs that have the potential to induce tachyarrhythmias, which may predispose the patient to a greater incidence of arrhythmia and increased mortality (Wilkoff, 2006; Wilkoff *et al.*, 2006).

The issue of inappropriate therapy is also a major concern for manufactures and health providers, as repeated shocks are known to promote further arrhythmia (Exner *et al.*, 2001; NICE, 2007; Pinski and Fahy, 1995; Wilkoff, 2006; Wilkoff *et al.*, 2006). Pashkow *et al.* (1997) performed an extensive review of the literature concerning exercise for patients with malignant arrhythmias and ICDs. The important points raised were as follows:

- ICDs predominantly assess rate, not rhythm, and that sinus tachycardia within the detection zone (sinus crossover) could be considered rapid and therapy delivered. The safeguard is that a certain number of beats (programmable) have to occur before action is taken by the ICD.
- Inappropriate therapies are uncomfortable at the very least and debilitating for some patients.
- Such therapy can lead to the induction or worsening of malignant arrhythmias.

Although some improvements have occurred, they are not necessarily addressing the areas of most concern (NICE, 2007; Wilkoff, 2006; Wilkoff *et al.*, 2006). These authors have found that dual-chamber devices tended to oversense ventricular and atrial activity and, although detected with considerable accuracy, the ICDs often failed to differentiate oversensing from arrhythmias and did not withhold therapy.

The frequency and reason for inappropriate therapy is quantifiable, as the device stores the rhythm history. Maron *et al.* (2000) found, in a study of 128 patients, that 32 (25%) of patients had inappropriate therapy and that 29 (23%) of patients had appropriate therapy. The authors concluded that the rate of inappropriate therapy was determined by the algorithms use; the single and dual programmability of the device and the reason for implantation.

A more recent clinical presentation that further confounds the ICD therapy issue is that in some instances ICD sensitivity leads to oversensing and results in a series of activity referred to as an 'electrical storm'. This is characterised by the occurrence of three or more shocks within a 24-hour period and represents a major issue for electrophysiologists and patients with ICDs. The evidence is developing for a strong relationship between these electrical storms and an increased risk of death (Exner *et al.*, 2001; Pinski and Fahy, 1995; Wilkoff, 2006). The authors considered whether the electrical storm played an inciting, contributing or bystander role in the increased mortality and concluded that presently the role was biased towards a contributing role. Elevated troponin (indicative of myocardial muscle damage), increased fibrosis and cellular injury following recent shocks are factors that lead to this decision. Interestingly, the authors close with a summary comment, suggesting that the increased relative risk of death was independent of known prognostic factors and LVEF. This suggests a dependent role for electrical storms and frequent ICD cardioversion/defibrillation shocks and is indicative of some causal effect on mortality.

Patient's experience of ICD therapy

Patient's experience of ICD therapy will vary according to programme settings:

Antitachycardia pacing for ventricular tachycardia, in which the patient may experience palpitations or be totally unaware that therapy has been delivered. Most patients report that pacing is perceived to be painless.

Cardioversion for fast ventricular tachycardia, in which a low- to moderate-energy shock is delivered which may be mildly uncomfortable, often described as a 'thump on the chest'.

Defibrillation for VF, in which a high-energy shock is delivered and has been described as a 'kick or heavy thump in the chest'.

Some patients have no warning signs before the device delivers therapy. Others experience dizziness, palpitations or lose consciousness. It must be remembered in VF that the patient may become unconscious very quickly due to loss of cardiac output, and once the device has recognised this abnormal rhythm it may take between 5 and 7 seconds to charge prior to firing.

Knowledge of patient's experiences of ICD therapy is important in terms of developing protocols to manage a patient who may report symptoms or lose consciousness during attendance at a CR programme.

Families and health care professionals may harbour worries that they too may experience the ICD device therapy when touching the patient at the time of shock. However, the strength of the shock is a maximum of 35 J, far less than that required for external defibrillation, and this energy diminishes as it travels through the body. Therefore, someone touching a patient at the time of shock will only feel a mild tingling sensation at most (i.e. 2 J).

Population characteristics of patients fitted with an ICD

Implantation selection criteria of post-MI, heart failure (NYHA classes II and III) and arrhythmic conditions produce considerable heterogeneity within the ICD population. The age range of patients fitted with ICDs incorporates both young and old, although the mean age derived from the combination of the ICD trials was 54 (SD 14). This value is biased due to the recruitment of only adults into the trials. The study by Maron *et al.* (2000) within 128 hypertrophic cardiomyopathy patients found a mean age of 40 (SD 16) and a range of 8–82. Sotile and Sears (1999) highlighted that within health care, a young patient was anyone under the age of 50 years, and that this was not helpful, since the issues faced by teenage ICD patients are very different to those faced by older patients. They use the phrase 'enduring loss' and suggest that the young ICD patients lose the naivety of being completely healthy, are conditioned to be cautious and have a dependency on the health care system.

With the differences highlighted, there remains one dramatic common denominator that unites most, if not all, ICD patients, namely they have either suffered or are very likely to suffer SCD episodes. This factor produces a unique psychological state that continues to be appreciated as the clinical burden increases.

Psychosocial and exercise behaviour issues

Namerow *et al.* (1999) assessed quality of life during the first 6 months of implantation. They compared 228 control patients from the CABG surgery only group with 262 patients that had CABG and ICDs. They used the SF-36 questionnaire and other psychosocial measures and found that the ICD patients had lower levels of psychological well-being compared to the controls. In addition, patients who had a shock delivered by the ICD reported even poorer well-being and had lower physical functioning. The assumption that natural recovery would ameliorate the distressed state cannot be supported within the ICD population (Namerow *et al.*, 1999).

Sotile and Sears (1999) have performed extensive work with ICD patients, partners, carers and clinical staff and produced a reference manual that clarifies many of the issues faced by all involved. Sotile and Sears (1999) estimate that the levels of anxiety are somewhere between 13 and 40%, reporting clinically significant levels. Lewin *et al.* (2001) reviewed the ICD literature with a psychological focus and suggest that over 30% of ICD patients have clinical states of anxiety and depression post-implant and that these can lead to behaviour adjustments that will reduce an individual's level of functioning.

Some patients can present to rehabilitation specialists as having a global fear of exercise, as they are not always aware of the electrical storm, but simply think they should not exercise (Sears *et al.*, 2001). Fear is a powerful stimulus and has profound physiological, psychological and emotional consequences that are associated with considerable behaviour adaptation. Over time and in association with antecedent avoidance behaviour, this can and does lead to a reduction in functional capacity (Lewin *et al.*, 2001; NICE, 2000; Sears *et al.*, 2001). Long-term exposure to this behaviour, if not addressed, can reduce a formerly independent person to a dependent state that may preclude activities as simple as walking. Continued attenuation of daily activities and avoidance of formal exercise for most ICD patients creates a downward spiral that can lead to considerable debilitation (Sotile and Sears, 1999). Patients can present with such low functional capacity that they are ineligible for rehabilitation, not solely because of the risk of sudden death; rather, they are in such poor physical condition that they could not exercise sufficiently even if they wished to. This has considerable emotional and psychological effects, with elevated anxiety, associated depression and a lack of confidence beyond the confines of their daily lives (Sotile and Sears, 1999). CR exercise professionals should be aware of these important and unique psychosocial issues when devising strategies to increase and maintain exercise behaviours in this group of patients. In addition to the extra psychological burden of ICDs, these patients will need continued support, behaviour change and maintenance. The CR exercise professionals will need all their experience and skills in maintaining healthy exercise behaviour (see more in Thow, 2006, Ch. 8).

Evidence for cardiac rehabilitation in high-risk patients

The team of Coats *et al.* (1992) and Davey *et al.* (1992) performed physiological studies on the effects of 8 weeks of exercise training on 17 and 22 male heart failure patients, respectively. Coat *et al.* (1992) detailed the intrinsic cardiac and haemodynamic findings and Davey *et al.* (1992) detailed the cardiorespiratory adaptation to training. Although there were criticisms of the study design, it should not detract from the strength of the studies, as they demonstrated cardiovascular and respiratory adaptation alongside improved performance in high-risk heart failure patients with associated low cardiac function (mean LVEF of 19.6%, SD 2.3).

The contribution of central (cardiac output) and peripheral (AVO_2 difference) components of VO_2max was important in this population, since it has been argued that the heart of a patient in failure is unlikely to adapt (Bowman *et al.*, 1998). Central adaptation occurred with an increase in stroke volume at submaximal exercise (25 W) and an increase in stroke volume and HR at peak exercise. The increase in stroke volume could be interpreted as an increased inotropic (myocardial muscle force) capacity, but could equally be considered a product of peripheral vascular adjustment in the form of greater preload and reduced afterload on the heart. Williams *et al.* (2001) acknowledge that the direct measurement of the inotropic capacity of the ventricles is very difficult, as the ventricles form one component of a highly complex pressure maintenance system. Evidence of this type reinforces the need to assess and manage these patients with exercise so that functional capacity (FC) and equivalent cardiac output can be maintained or increased.

Left ventricular ejection fraction and function relationship

Many authors have suggested that patients with the lowest FC have the most to gain (Bethell, 1996; Blair *et al.*, 1995; Fleg *et al.*, 2000). Large-scale evidence of this came from Blair *et al.* (1995) with a prospective study of change in physical activity status on mortality and morbidity. They found that patients with the lowest FC and sedentary status that subsequently changed to moderate activity had the greatest improvement in FC and greatest reduction in mortality. Balady *et al.* (1996) performed a study on CHD patients with a wide range of LVEF and FC. The population were categorised into two groups: low FC (<5 METs, $N = 163$) and high FC (>5 METs). Both categories of patients made significant gains in FC post-rehabilitation, and further to this the low category patients gained significantly more than those in the high FC category. The work of Fitchet *et al.* (2003) (Figure 4.6) found a similar tendency, in that patients with an LVEF of 20% could make greater than 1.2 METs gain whereas those with 55% LVEF may only make 0.5 METs gain.

Bowman *et al.* (1998) reviewed the literature regarding CR for heart failure patients and concluded that exclusion from CR exercise is common with poor LVEF and low FC and an increased risk of SCD being considered as the main exclusion criteria. Patients with low capacity and poor haemodynamics were assumed not to improve from CR exercise, and it was assumed that exacerbation of the condition could ensue. Bowman *et al.* (1998) did, however, highlight the benefits for heart failure patients who were considered fit enough to attend CR. The gains, they argue, were mainly a consequence of peripheral adaptations, with increased economy

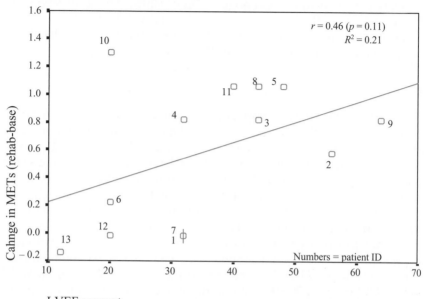

Figure 4.6 Ejection fractions and function relationship (Fitchet *et al.*, 2003).

and improved lactic acid tolerance seen as the primary mechanisms for improvement.

Arrhythmia risk in context

There are continued reminders in the media and to a degree in the scientific literature about how risky exercise is with regard to sudden death, but on closer inspection the context for arrhythmia is unclear. The following include some of the views on the issue:

• Heart attacks occur during or soon after exercise, and the risk increases in persons who do not exercise regularly (Pina *et al.*, 2003).

• Approximately 5–10% of heart attacks are associated with vigorous physical activity (Thompson *et al.*, 2007).

• Vigorous exercise training is not associated with prevalence of ventricular arrhythmias in elderly athletes (Pigozzi *et al.*, 2004).

• Exercise can induce or prevent arrhythmias: it depends how you do it (Beckerman *et al.*, 2005).

• People with cardiac disease are seven times more likely to die suddenly during sedentary activities than during jogging (Thompson *et al.*, 2007).

• Cardiac monitoring of daily activity confirms that most arrhythmias occur at rest or during sedentary activity (Pina *et al.*, 2003; Thompson *et al.*, 2007).

• Arrhythmia can only be induced by exercise in approximately 14% of patients with known arrhythmogenic right ventricular cardiomyopathy (Corrado et al., 2001).
• Cardiac patients are more likely to have arrhythmias during sleep than during moderate-intensity exercise (Thompson et al., 2007).

Evidence for CR exercise training in ICD patients

Exercise training in the ICD population is minimal to non-existent in the literature, with only the occasional empirical reference from individual case studies. The most extensive literature reviews to date were by Pashkow et al. (1997) and Lampman and Knight (2000) who considered exercise for patients with arrhythmia and ICDs. They found no evidence of comprehensive CR, and this was reiterated in the NICE (2000) guidelines, which acknowledged that a rehabilitative approach including exercise should be developed and evaluated for ICD patients.

The first prospective randomised control trial in ICD patients with low capacity (LVEF <35%) demonstrated that exercise-based rehabilitation has significant and beneficial outcomes in terms of FC and psychological well-being (Fitchet et al., 2003). The finding of a 20% mean improvement in FC following exercise training was similar to the earlier work and was achieved without the need for ECG monitoring during exercise.

Vanhees et al. (2001) performed a retrospective study on a group of 8 ICD patients going through a rehabilitation programme (exercise-based) and matched them with patients who were comparable for age, sex, body mass index, LVEF and duration of the programme. Mean ejection fraction was 44% (SD 10). This represents a high percentage of ejection fraction for ICD patients, especially compared to the risk classification criteria and implantation criteria (<35%) quoted previously (NICE, 2000). This study concluded that ICD patients could perform exercise safely.

Frizelle et al. (2004) surveyed all UK ICD implantation centres with the aim of highlighting ICD patients' needs. Of the respondents, 99% stated that CR should be offered to ICD patients, but only 36% did so. All centres that did not offer CR believed that the needs of their patients were not being met. This survey demonstrated that specialist centres considered that CR would meet the needs of their patients, but access was poor. CR services should be more inclusive of ICD patients as they are ideal to meet their needs, as ICD patients have similar needs to long-term cardiac patients (Lewin et al., 2001).

Why CR for an ICD patient?

The implantation selection criteria, particularly MADITT II, show that the majority of patients with an ICD have some degree of ischaemic heart disease, for which the benefits of CR with exercise training are well documented (Vanhees *et al.*, 2004). ICD patients have a reduced functional capacity, enhanced by a fear of arrhythmia, SCD and inappropriate therapy on exercise (Begley *et al.*, 2003; Luthje *et al.*, 2005). Avoidance behaviour with previous shocks may exist, for example avoidance of walking to the shops. The greatest fears for patients are the effects of the device firing or the anticipation of firing. Ninety per cent of individuals are shown to assign a cause for the device therapy, and assigning a cause leads to a progressively restricted lifestyle. Such behaviour is likely to create a downward spiral of activity levels.

High levels of clinical anxiety and depression exist in ICD patients, as much as 40% clinical anxiety and 30% clinical depression (Sears *et al.*, 1999). CR with psychological support has been shown to be effective in reducing both anxiety and depression.

The ICD is designed to provide immediate emergency treatment rather than constricting activity due to fear that activity will provoke an arrhythmia. Return to regular physical activity should be promoted, as improvement in functional capacity in turn improves parasympathetic tone and heart rate variability, thereby reducing arrhythmia risk (Belardinelli, 2003; Malfatto *et al.*, 1996; Pigozzi *et al.*, 2004).

Lewin *et al.* (2001) critically reviewed the CR literature and concluded that ICD patients have similar needs to those of chronic cardiac patients. CR is the ideal template to address the needs of ICD patients.

Service drivers for ICD and rehabilitation

There are many service drivers for the inclusion of ICD patients in CR services, as shown in Box 4.2. Thus, exercise professionals should be prepared to include patients with ICDs into all phases of CR.

Box 4.2 Service drivers for ICD and rehabilitation.

1. NSF for CHD: Chapter 6 (HF), Chapter 7 (CR), Chapter 8 (Arrhythmia and Sudden Cardiac Death)
2. NSF for long-term conditions
3. SIGN guideline (no. 57)
4. BACR guidelines
5. NICE 2000 ICD guidelines (no. 11) 'A rehabilitative approach to aftercare which includes psychological preparation for living with an ICD.'
6. BHF: Heart failure programmes
7. Cochrane reviews in favour exercise-based CR
8. DH: Choosing health – physical activity plan
9. NHS staff as champions of health promotion

Cardiac rehabilitation assessment

The CR exercise leaders must remember that it is not the ICD that they are treating, but the underlying cardiac status and function of the patient which is the primary consideration. Assessment should follow the usual process as for other cardiac patients, with particular consideration of the following:
- Cardiac function
- Risk stratification
- ICD device thresholds and settings
- Shock history and any related avoidance behaviours
- β-Blockade dose
- Perceived limitations of lifestyle

For all services that include ICD patients in the rehabilitation process, it is advised that communication links and referral routes are established with the electrophysiology team to discuss any concerns.

Prior to embarking on any form of physical activity with the patient, it is essential that there is information on current device thresholds and therapy settings, so that the relationship of the target heart rate can be made with the device thresholds.

The important points that need consideration prior to prescribing exercise or giving advice on physical activity are as follows:
1. The ICD detection threshold setting in beats per minute
2. Whether the device is set for VT or VF
3. Rapid onset and sustained VT settings
4. ICD therapy, for example, antitachycardia pacing or shocks
5. Use and dose of β-blockade

Significance of the ICD threshold in the exercise prescription

The relationship between ICD and exercise training thresholds (Table 4.6) is of importance to practitioners. The choice of 75% maximum is based on previous studies on high-risk patients (Coats *et al.*, 1992; Pashkow *et al.*, 1997). The recommendation to keep the exercise HR 10 beats below ICD detection threshold is not always easy and casts doubt on the use of age-adjusted maximum heart rate (AAMHR) in this population, as found by Fitchet *et al.* (2003). For instance, one patient (ID 11, Table 4.6) is at risk from this approach and one other (ID 13, Table 4.6) where HR would quickly be within the detection zone. The patient (ID 13, Table 4.6) was of particular consideration due to the lack of chronotropic constraint, as β-blockade was not prescribed due to heart failure.

There are five other patients in Table 4.6, where the 75% target is less than 20% away from their ICD detection lower limit. As stated earlier, it is not inevitable that the ICD will interpret sinus tachycardia as an arrhythmia whilst in the detection zone. However, sinus tachycardia can be

Table 4.6 Target heart rate and ICD detection for each patient.

Patient ID	75% AAMHR	ICD detection	THR % of ICD detection	Rhythm	Response	LVEF %	β-Blockade
1	129	150	86	VT	ATP	30	Nil
2	119	150	80	VT	ATP	55	Nil
3	117	188	62	VF	Shock	45	β-Blockade
4	124	194	64	VF	Shock	30	Nil
5	119	200	60	VF	Shock	49	Nil
6	126	150	84	VT	ATP	20	β-Blockade
7	112	136	82	VT	ATP	30	β-Blockade
8	111	158	70	VT	ATP	42	β-Blockade
9	121	188	64	VF	Shock	65	β-Blockade
10	116	164	70	VT	ATP	20	Nil
11	140	100	140	VT	ATP	40	β-Blockade
12	118	140	84	VT	ATP	20	β-Blockade
13	121	125	97	VT	ATP	12	Nil
14	125	188	67	VF	Shock	35	β-Blockade
15	117	176	66	VF	Shock	70	β-Blockade
16	134	200	67	VF	Shock	40	β-Blockade

Note: ICD detection threshold and target heart rate (THR) = 75% AAMHR.

misinterpreted and cross over in this situation. Given the physical and psychological implications of dealing with a shock and the long-term issues with inappropriate ICD therapies, a proactive approach to avoiding this situation is considered best practice (Exner *et al.*, 2001; Pinski and Fahy, 1995; Wilkoff, 2006).

Many ICD patients will be taking β-blockade, which in terms of exercise safety creates a degree of comfort. The benefits of β-blockade in keeping heart rates down are evident in the exercise test results of 5445 referred cardiac patients using the Bruce protocol (Table 4.7). Patients can achieve at least the same amount of work for less haemodynamic response. For patients that are set on slow VT (e.g. 120–150 beats/min) β-blockade use can contribute significantly to the lowering of myocardial demand during normal daily functioning.

To further improve the safety of exercising this population, the stratification of each individual for an arrhythmia or other cardiac event during exercise must be considered. The majority of patients who have been implanted with an ICD would be classified as high risk according to traditional risk stratification (AACVPR, 2006; ACSM, 2006a). For high-risk individuals it would be prudent to reduce the intensity of the exercise prescription to the lower target for moderate-intensity exercise (60–80% AAMHR or 50–70% heart rate reserve (HRR)), that is 60% when using AAMHR equations and 50% of HRR.

Figure 4.7 shows conceptually how the ICD monitors exercise heart rate. A knowledge of these factors and their interrelationship can reduce

Table 4.7 Exercise test outcome in association to β-blockade use.

β-Blockade	METs	Peak HR	RPP
Not prescribed			
Mean	9	158	283
SD	3	22	55
N	3724	3724	3724
Stopped for ET			
Mean	8	157	288
SD	3	21	55
N	978	978	978
Continued for ET			
Mean	9	124	212
SD	3	20	50
N	743	743	743

METs, metabolic equivalents; RPP, rate pressure product; ET, exercise test.

the anxiety of patients and clinicians involved in setting physical activity and exercise targets. The ICD threshold (see Figure 4.7) (1) is determined by the electrophysiologist at implant and is the point at which arrhythmia can be induced by electrical stimulation. It is imperative that exercise heart rate is kept below this level. The ICD compares the ECG shape (2) from one heartbeat to the next and retains a memory of the ECG profiles associated with previous arrhythmias. Rapid onset (3) and stability over time (4) criteria enable the ICD to discriminate between sinus tachycardia and true arrhythmias and can be adjusted by a cardiac physiologist, with the

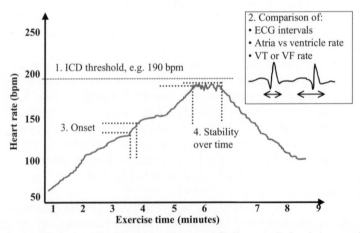

Figure 4.7 Schematic view of implantable cardioverter defibrillator monitoring during exercise.

aid of device-specific software, after implantation. Collectively these criteria are effective at reducing inappropriate therapy.

Exercise testing in ICD patients

When patients are asked to exercise as part of an assessment procedure or treatment, there is a need to be vigilant for sudden changes in their haemodynamics and rhythm. This is especially so if a patient has low FC, known arrhythmia or associated heart failure, as the risk of SCD in this population is higher than in any other group (Beckerman *et al.*, 2005; Belardinelli, 2003; Coats *et al.*, 1992; Pashkow *et al.*, 1997). One of the main issues relates to the choice of maximum versus submaximum and functional tests and what best fits with the needs of patients (Doherty, 2006; Fitchet *et al.*, 2003; Lampman and Knight, 2000; Pashkow *et al.*, 1997).

Pinski and Fahy (1995) reviewed the literature and found conclusive evidence that maximum and submaximum exercise testing provokes arrhythmias or ICD discharge and recommend that the programmed detection interval of the device should be known before testing. If the device has been implanted for VF or fast VT, this rate will normally exceed that attained during exercise-induced sinus tachycardia, and the test or exercise can be terminated as the heart rate approaches 10 beats/min below the detection interval of the device. The authors acknowledge the use of deactivation procedures (magnet or programmed) and suggest that these procedures ensure a degree of safety from inappropriate, unpleasant and potentially hazardous shocks. Within their review they acknowledge that on occasions the use of a magnet can actually evoke ICD therapy, especially ATP, and acts as pro-arrhythmia that can develop to full arrhythmia. They suggest that high-level technical support is necessary for deactivation via programming.

General, rather than patient-specific exercise test or training protocols are evident in the literature and contribute to this view (Lampman and Knight, 2000). Pinski and Fahy (1995) suggest that traditional exercise testing protocols that incorporate simultaneous increases in speed and gradient contribute to the high rate of inappropriate therapy due to sinus tachycardia crossover. It is, therefore, recommended that in patients who are at a high risk of an arrhythmia, the ETT does not produce such a haemodynamic challenge from tests such as the Bruce protocol and that only one parameter, that is speed or gradient should be used to increase the exercise intensity at any time.

The work of Fitchet *et al.* (2003) showed that the exercise test should reflect the ability of the patient and have default characteristics, such as a warm-up component, single incremental progression and a cool-down phase, that are associated with a reduced likelihood of arrhythmia. Many of the functional tests used in conventional CR are highly appropriate as they incorporate these features.

Exercise programme design

The design of exercise programmes is an area of extensive research, and the literature offers many different approaches to make the process safe and effective. The consensus suggests that the frequency, intensity, timing and type of exercise are the primary determinants of the exercise training effect (ACSM, 2006a; Åstrand *et al.*, 2003; Heyward, 2002; McArdle *et al.*, 2001). These factors have been conceptualised as the FITT principle (Fletcher *et al.*, 2001; Heyward, 2002). In addition, it is believed that an 'E' for Enjoyment should always be incorporated into the principle, that is FITTE.

Specificity of training

CR exercise circuits routinely have an aerobic theme and callisthenic exercises similar to movements encountered in daily activities (Bethell, 1996; Bethell *et al.*, 2001). The use of functional exercise has long been considered important, so that the conditioning effect occurs in the muscles used during daily activities. This approach is in part related to the arteriovenous oxygen difference (AVO_2 difference) and the fact that the muscles used during exercise demonstrate change and improved efficiency (Richardson, 2000). If the activity is functional then the gains achieved from training are considered to have the greatest carryover to daily life. Many authors have highlighted the relationship between training and extent of carryover into subsequent activity (Durstine and Davis, 2001; McCafferty and Hovarth, 1977; Saltin *et al.*, 1976).

The term 'specificity of training' conceptualised this phenomenon and Saltin *et al.* (1976) and McCafferty and Hovarth (1977) published what seems to be the earliest articles on this concept. Collectively, they suggest that training adaptations are specific to the cells and their structural and physiological processes, and that the nature of the stimulus determines the extent of adaptability. In other words, exercise stress is relative and selective, and elicits specific adaptation and specific training effects.

Although there are many aspects to specificity, three fundamental principles need to be borne in mind when designing an exercise programme to enhance and maintain functional capacity:
1. Individual needs
2. Reversibility
3. Test specificity

The *individual needs* principle suggests that the subsequent utilisation of any training effect is minimal in activities that use different movements to those used in training. Although central cardiorespiratory adaptations occur in the delivery of blood to the active muscles following moderate exercise training, the major adaptation occurs in relation to the muscle type, energy pathways and muscle action utilised to perform the activity (ACSM, 2006a; McArdle *et al.*, 2001). These are specific and explain why other muscles, energy pathways and different muscle actions do not demonstrate the performance gain (Saltin *et al.*, 1976).

The *reversibility* principle relates to the deconditioning or detraining effect that accompanies a cessation of exercise training. The work of McArdle *et al.* (2001) suggests that a 25% decrease in VO_2max can occur within 20 days of stopping training and adopting a sedentary lifestyle.

Test specificity relates to the fact that the improved AVO_2 difference that accompanies training occurs in the muscles used for the activity (Richardson *et al.*, 2000). The carryover from training to different activities could be as little as 25% of the gains that a person acquired during training (McArdle *et al.*, 2001). Running seems to give the greatest carryover to alternative activities, with cycling and walking programmes leading to more peripheral adaptation (Durstine and Davis, 2001; McCafferty and Hovarth, 1977).

The importance of efficiency

Many patients with heart failure and low-capacity patients fitted with an ICD will benefit more in terms of efficiency than peak fitness (Fitchet *et al.*, 2003). The relationship between LVEF and potential improvement in exercise capacity is poor (Figure 4.6) (Fitchet *et al.*, 2003).

Figure 4.8 shows the results from 11 ICD patients from a controlled trial and demonstrates that patients can achieve slightly more exercise for

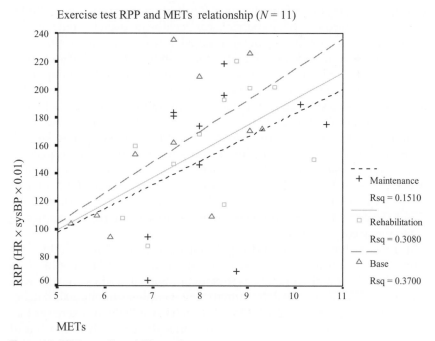

Figure 4.8 Efficiency effect of CR exercise.

less overall demand on the cardiovascular system as measured by rate–pressure product.

Type of exercise

An exercise intensity greater than 50% of maximum capacity has been agreed as the minimum for healthy subjects and mild-to-moderate cardiac disease patients, and an intensity of 40% has been found to be effective in the more severely affected cardiac patients (ACSM, 2006a; Blair *et al.*, 2004; Coats *et al.*, 1992). There is a dose–response relationship between the frequency and intensity of exercise prescription, whereby the most favourable fitness improvements occur with hard-intensity, high-frequency exercise, followed by moderate-intensity, high-frequency and hard-intensity, low-frequency exercises (Duncan *et al.*, 2005; Lee *et al.*, 2003). One major contribution to our understanding came from a complex randomised trial of intensity and frequency in 492 sedentary, healthy men and women who used walking as the primary intervention (Duncan *et al.*, 2005). Although the work has some methodological flaws in respect of sampling and variation in the volume of exercise across the five test conditions, it nevertheless showed that significant improvement in fitness (10% increase in FC) and improved lipid profile could be achieved and maintained over 2 years, with walking as the mode of exercise.

The physical demands of the patients' daily life in terms of aerobic demand, muscular strength, endurance, flexibility and coordination should be taken into account so that patients can feel the greatest benefit (ACSM, 2006a; Coats *et al.*, 1995). Aerobic and skilled flowing movement, efficiency, muscular strength, endurance and flexibility should dominate the exercise and physical activity sessions. The need for specific strength training stems from the evidence that suggests that aerobic exercise alone does not lead to increased muscle strength, although strength training does have a beneficial effect on aerobic fitness (Durstine and Davis, 2001; McArdle *et al.*, 2001).

In many respects, strength assessment and training should be key CR exercise components. A reduction in activities of daily living, especially in the elderly, can soon lead to a concomitant reduction in strength and wasting of skeletal muscle tissue associated with poor heart function and reduced quality of life (Latham *et al.*, 2003). Avoidance of muscle atrophy should be a primary goal, followed by an increase in strength, if appropriate to the needs of the patient.

It appears both logical and highly effective to combine aerobic and strength/endurance training. Activities used in the circuit should be as close to those of daily function as reasonable. Such activities are very well tolerated, effective and lead to optimal carryover (Belardinelli, 2003; Fitchet *et al.*, 2003; Fletcher *et al.*, 2001; Pina *et al.*, 2003). Callisthenic exercises that closely match functional activities also reduce the risk of ICD shock lead problems, which are thought to be associated with excessive range and/or highly repetitive shoulder movements (Fitchet *et al.*, 2003; Lampman and Knight, 2000; Pashkow *et al.*, 1997; Pina *et al.*, 2003).

Design of the exercise circuit

Group exercise and circuit training, although not for everyone, are highly effective in rehabilitation, as they enable individuals to follow their own prescription of exercise whilst sharing that experience with others. This approach is the mode of CR throughout the UK (Bethell *et al.*, 2001) and is endorsed in the NSF for CHD (DH, 2005) and the ACPICR (2006) as a viable solution to the increasing numbers of patients who now access CR.

CR programme design is such that it reduces the risk of arrhythmia or cardiac events, which are the primary risks for all cardiac patients during exercise. These include the following:
• Risk stratification with associated reduced intensity within the moderate range for high-risk patients
• Appropriate functional assessment from which to set an exercise prescription
• Prolonged incremental warm-up
• Monitoring including HR, BP, RPP, rate of perceived exertion (RPE) and good observation
• Prolonged decreasing cool-down

The CR exercise programme design is therefore suited to ICD patients, with the additional knowledge of ICD threshold and relationship to target heart rate, with appropriate use of exercise monitoring.

An example of an exercise circuit based on earlier work (Fitchet *et al.*, 2003) is shown in Figure 4.9. The exercises are made more demanding by

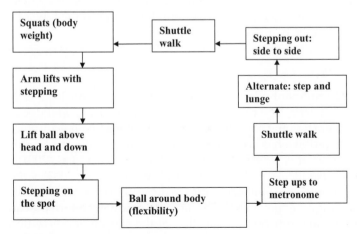

Figure 4.9 CR exercise circuit content example.

altering the range of movement, cadence, duration and, where appropriate, load.

ICD lead problems

Caution is required with those few patients who are at risk of lead failure. This situation often occurs immediately postoperatively and exists because the only viable route to the ventricle required the ICD lead to bend or twist slightly more than normal. It is important to be extra vigilant with these patients and avoid excessive shoulder range of movement and/or highly repetitive vigorous shoulder movements (Fitchet *et al.*, 2003; Lampman and Knight, 2000; Pashkow *et al.*, 1997; Pina *et al.*, 2003). Light- to moderate-resistance activities performed within a normal range of movement, which closely match functional activities, have been used successfully in patients with an ICD (Fitchet *et al.*, 2003).

Warm-up

Warm-up is crucial for properly preparing cardiovascular and musculoskeletal systems to meet the demands of exercise and avoiding complications (ACSM, 2006a, b; Belardinelli, 2003; Fletcher *et al.*, 2001; Pina *et al.*, 2003; Vincent *et al.*, 2003). The evidence suggests that warm-up should be incremental and normally last between 10 and 15 minutes. One of the most important aspects of warm-up, in low-capacity patients, is avoidance of severe breathlessness. At the point when severe breathlessness occurs, the cardiovascular system shunts the blood (oxygen) supply to the accessory muscle of respiration, which results in a 15% relative loss in oxygen consumption by the active skeletal muscle (Richardson, 2000; Richardson *et al.*, 2000). Movements should be free ranging, encourage gradual extensibility of the muscles and be similar to the type of activity performed in the main exercise overload session.

Cool-down

The most important advice to give patients about exercise is *not to suddenly stop exercise.* The risk of cardiac complications is well documented shortly after stopping an exercise, especially in the first few minutes, and a graded cool-down has been found to reduce the incidence (ACSM, 2006a, b; Beckerman *et al.*, 2005; Belardinelli, 2003; Fletcher *et al.*, 2001; Mayordomo and Batalla, 2002; Pina *et al.*, 2003; Vincent *et al.*, 2003). Cool-down exercise should use similar activities to those in the warm-up, but with less force and range of movement. The aim is to gradually return the cardiorespiratory system function to near that of the starting levels within 10–15 minutes (ACSM, 2006a, b; Belardinelli, 2003; Fletcher *et al.*, 2001; Pina *et al.*, 2003; Vincent *et al.*, 2003).

Conditioning component

The main part of the training programme should consist of graded aerobic circuit training. The aim is for patients to achieve a minimum of 20 minutes of continuous cardiovascular exercise and up to 40 minutes, incorporating multi-joint movements with body weight and moderate resistance (ACSM, 2006a; Duncan *et al.*, 2005; Fitchet *et al.*, 2003; Fletcher *et al.*, 2001; Lampman and Knight, 2000; Pashkow *et al.*, 1997).

For the low-functioning patients, cardiovascular exercise should be alternated with active rest stations in order to achieve the exercise prescription time. As the patient improves in efficiency, the active rest should be gradually replaced by a cardiovascular exercise in order to achieve the goal of 20 minutes minimum continuous state. This sequence of arm exercise followed by legwork, with flexibility and coordination exercises following the more strenuous exercise, enables participants to better endure the session, thus avoiding local muscle ache, a factor that can lead to premature cessation of exercise (ACSM, 2006a; Coats *et al.*, 1995; Heyward, 2002). Feet should be kept moving during active rest to ensure venous return and to counteract pooling and the potential for hypotension.

Exercises in standing or sitting?

In general, most exercises should be performed in standing, with horizontal and seated arm exercises kept to a minimum. Seated arm exercise is associated with reduced venous return, reduced end-diastolic volume, a concomitant decrease in cardiac output and increased likelihood of arrhythmia (Fitchet *et al.*, 2003; Lampman and Knight, 2000; Pashkow *et al.*, 1997). If seated exercise is to be performed then the intensity of exercise should be lowered and the emphasis placed on muscular endurance. Perform exercises in standing. Even though based on a low level of evidence, mild leg exercise, for example alternate leg movements, when combined with arm exercise is thought to reduce venous return compared with strict arm work alone (Toner *et al.*, 1990). The age, ability, extent of cardiomyopathy and heart failure within ICD patients rule out patients moving from floor exercise to standing exercise. Finally, floor exercises such as sit-ups have limited functional cardiovascular benefits. If using floor exercise, these should be at the end of the cardiovascular section to avoid patients repeatedly moving from floor to standing.

Breathing and isometric muscle work

Breath holding and sustained isometric muscle work are associated with reduced venous return, reduced end-diastolic volume, a concomitant decrease in cardiac output and increased likelihood of arrhythmia. Isometric work, particularly of the abdominal region, should be avoided especially during arm exercise in patients with low FC (AACVPR, 2006; ACSM,

2006a; Lampman and Knight, 2000; Lee *et al.*, 2003; Pashkow *et al.*, 1997; Pina *et al.*, 2003; Vincent *et al.*, 2003).

Additional considerations for safe exercise prescription in patients with an ICD are as follows:
1. Perform exercises in standing
2. Avoid breath holding
3. Limit sustained isometric work especially of abdomen

Patient monitoring

Exercise prescription should utilise one of the evidence-based approaches of monitoring, for example RPE or heart rate reserve. Caution is required when prescribing exercise intensity based on standard heart rate approaches. The use of 75% AAMHR in patients with slow VT will often mean that the target heart rate is above the detection threshold of the ICD. This can be avoided by using HRR (Fitchet *et al.*, 2003). Sinus tachycardia is a normal response to exercise, and although most modern ICDs have algorithms designed to differentiate sinus from ventricular tachyarrhythmias, there are still occasions when inappropriate therapy is administered (Begley *et al.*, 2003; Luthje *et al.*, 2005). Every effort should be made to reduce patient anxiety in regard to perceived physical activity and exercise risks, in order to achieve the best outcome post-implant (Lewin *et al.*, 2001; Sears *et al.*, 2001).

Telemetry HR monitoring and polar monitoring are safe to use and help staff and patients keep the exercise HR 10 beats below ICD detection threshold, as recommended (Fitchet *et al.*, 2003; Pinski and Fahy, 1995). A stethoscope and manual sphygmomanometer are essential equipment, and we recommend them above the automated versions for use during the CR exercise programme. Both telemetry HR and BP monitoring are reliable in these groups (Fitchet *et al.*, 2003), and HR measurement has an absolute error of 4 (SD 5.2) beats/min.

Maintenance of the CR training effect

The attainment of a new level of fitness requires that training be continued at a level sufficient to maintain the effect. This is generally agreed and evident in polices that guide exercise training as an intervention to promote health. Phase IV rehabilitation and long-term physical activity of the UK government's assurance framework for exercise referral systems (DH, 2007) are prime examples of the need to continue with a level of exercise or physical activity as part of a way of life. The reason for this is that the benefits of training are quickly lost, and research over many years has shown this to be the case.

The rate of loss of a recently acquired training effect is relative to the extent of FC. Patients with low FC levels have demonstrated as much as a 100% reduction in performance within 10 weeks of stopping rehabilitation

(ACSM, 2006a). Maintenance of a lower level of exercise intensity following rehabilitation is associated with a decreased rate of loss of the training effect (Fletcher *et al.*, 2001), and this can enable the benefits of exercise to exist for a longer period. The intensity of exercise, rather than the duration or frequency, has the greatest impact on the maintenance of FC (ACSM, 2006a). Maintenance of existing levels of physical fitness is relative to the initial level of activity. Recently acquired FC gains would easily be reduced to pre-training levels if the gains are not utilised by the individual during daily activities. This reiterates the needs principle of training specificity; if you do not use the activity, you will lose the ability.

The BACR phase 4 certificate, which qualifies exercise instructors to adapt and prescribe safe and effective exercise programmes to cardiac patients, is now inclusive of ICD patients. CR exercise professionals should work closely with their local BACR exercise providers to ensure referral and access to leisure facilities for ICD patients to continue their exercise training.

Specific physical activity and exercise advice for patients with an ICD

Exercise in water is safe but should be accompanied. Water-based activity will be similar for those with congestive heart failure. Thus, consideration of cardiac function should be made before advising water-based activities due to the detrimental haemodynamic effects of immersion in patients with a low LVEF.

Contact sports and aggressive movements with the arms need to be reduced and in some cases avoided where lead problems are known to exist.

Driving

A particularly worrying consequence of ICD therapy is that the UK Driving and Vehicle Licensing Agency (DVLA) will initially ban driving until the arrhythmia is under control. Patients have to request the return of licence and produce evidence from consultant cardiologists that the condition is stable. The ICD therapy rate per patient is checked annually by hospital returns to the DVLA, and any patient with two ICD shocks after implantation will have a further ban (DVLA, 2001). Patients are reluctant to do any activity that could potentially induce arrhythmia and ICD therapy, and it is imperative that exercise professionals keep this consequence in mind when setting the intensity of exercise.

Key messages

- We will see more patients with ICDs eligible for exercise-based CR.
- All patients with ICDs should be included in CR programmes.

- Physical activity and exercise have a substantial role in enabling patients to take control of their condition.
- Patients with an ICD can exercise safely without increasing the risk of cardiac complications.
- Information required prior to advising on activity:
  ○ ICD detection threshold setting in beats per minute
  ○ Device setting: VT or VF
  ○ Device onset and sustained VT settings
  ○ ICD therapy, for example antitachycardia pacing or shocks
  ○ Use and dose of β-blockade
- The mode of exercise needs to be similar to daily activity in order to gain most from training and maintain the effect over the long term.
- A long-term, preferably lifestyle, approach to physical activity and exercise is essential if patients are to achieve the greatest benefits.

Summary and conclusions

The evidence that this group of patients can gain substantial psychosocially, quality of life and physical fitness improvement is growing rapidly. Exercise professionals working in CR will, in future, have more patients with ICDs referred to their exercise classes. With an increased knowledge and understanding of the ICDs practitioners can ensure that these patients are given individualised exercise prescription that are safe and effective. The main challenge for the exercise professional is to help the patient overcome the fear and anxiety associated with exercise and arrhythmia and to make the most of life now they have the device.

References

Abraham, W.T., Fisher, W.G., Smith, A.L., *et al.* (2002) Cardiac resynchronization in chronic heart failure. *New England Journal of Medicine*, 346, 1845–53.

Ainsworth, B.E., Haskell, W.L., Leon, A.S., *et al.* (1993) Compendium of physical activities: classification of energy costs of human physical activities. *Medicine and Science in Sports and Exercise*, 25, 71–80.

American Association of Cardiovascular and Pulmonary Rehabilitation (AACVPR) (2006) *Guidelines for Cardiac Rehabilitation and Secondary Prevention Programs*, 7th edn. Champaign, IL: Human Kinetics.

American College of Sports Medicine (ACSM) (2006a) *Guidelines for Exercise Testing and Prescription*. Baltimore, MD: Lippincott Williams & Wilkins.

American College of Sports Medicine (ACSM) (2006b) *Resource Manual for Guidelines for Exercise Testing and Prescription*. Baltimore, MD: Lippincott Williams & Wilkins.

Association of Chartered Physiotherapists in Cardiac Rehabilitation (ACPICR) (2006) *Standards for the Exercise Component of Phase III Cardiac Rehabilitation*. London: CSP.

Åstrand, P., Rodahl, K., Dahl, H., *et al.* (2003) *Text Book of Work Physiology: Physiological Bases of Exercise.* Champaign, IL: Human Kinetics.

Balady, G.J., Jette, D., Scheer, J., *et al.* (1996) Changes in exercise capacity following cardiac rehabilitation in patients stratified according to age and gender. Results of the Massachusetts Association of Cardiovascular and Pulmonary Rehabilitation Multicenter Database. *Journal of Cardiopulmonary Rehabilitation,* 16, 38–46.

Beckerman, J., Wu, T., Jones, S., *et al.* (2005) Exercise test-induced arrhythmias. *Progress in Cardiovascular Disease,* 47, 285–305.

Begley, D.A., Mohiddin, S.A., Tripodi, D., *et al.* (2003) Efficacy of implantable cardioverter defibrillator therapy for primary and secondary prevention of sudden cardiac death in hypertrophic cardiomyopathy. *Pacing and Clinical Electrophysiology,* 26, 1887–96.

Belardinelli, R. (2003) Arrhythmias during acute and chronic exercise in chronic heart failure. *International Journal of Cardiology,* 90, 213–18.

Bethell, H. (1996) *Exercise-Based Cardiac Rehabilitation.* Kent, UK: Publishing Initiatives Books.

Bethell, H.J., Turner, S.C., Evans, J.A., *et al.* (2001) Cardiac rehabilitation in the United Kingdom. How complete is the provision? *Journal of Cardiopulmonary Rehabilitation,* 21, 111–15.

Blair, S.N., Kohl, H.W., III, Barlow, C.E., *et al.* (1995) Changes in physical fitness and all-cause mortality. A prospective study of healthy and unhealthy men. *Journal of the American Medical Association,* 273, 1093–8.

Blair, S.N., Lamonte, M.J., Nichaman, M.Z. (2004) The evolution of physical activity recommendations: how much is enough? *American Journal of Clinical Nutrition,* 79, 913S–20S.

Bowman, G.S., Thompson, D.R., Lewin R.J. (1998) Why are patients with heart failure not routinely offered cardiac rehabilitation. *Coronary Health Care,* 2, 187–92.

Braith, R.W., Edwards, D.G. (2003) Neurohormonal abnormalities in heart failure: impact of exercise training. *Congestive Heart Failure,* 9, 70–76.

Bryant, J., Brodin, H., Loveman, E., *et al.* (2005) The clinical and cost-effectiveness of implantable cardioverter defibrillators: a systematic review. *Health Technology Assessment,* 9, 1–150, iii.

Coats, A., Mcgee, H., Stokes, H., *et al.* (1995) *BACR Guidelines for Cardiac Rehabilitation.* London: Blackwell Science.

Coats, A.J., Adamopoulos, S., Radaelli, A., *et al.* (1992) Controlled trial of physical training in chronic heart failure. Exercise performance, hemodynamics, ventilation, and autonomic function. *Circulation,* 85, 2119–31.

Connolly, S.J., Gent, M., Roberts, R.S., *et al.* (2000) Canadian implantable defibrillator study (CIDS): a randomized trial of the implantable cardioverter defibrillator against amiodarone. *Circulation,* 101, 1297–302.

Corrado, D., Basso, C., Buja, G., *et al.* (2001) Right bundle branch block, right precordial ST-segment elevation, and sudden death in young people. *Circulation,* 103, 710–17.

Curtis, A.B., Cannom, D.S., Bigger, J.T., *et al.* (1997) Baseline characteristics of patients in the coronary artery bypass graft (CABG) patch trial. *American Heart Journal,* 134, 787–98.

Davey, P., Meyer, T., Coats, A., *et al.* (1992) Ventilation in chronic heart failure: effects of physical training. *British Heart Journal,* 68, 473–7.

Department of Health (DH) (2007) Department of health statement on exercise referral, London: HMSO, London, Crown copyright.

Department of Health (DH) (2005) Arrhythmias and sudden cardiac death. In: *National Service Framework for Coronary Heart Disease*. London: HMSO, London, Crown copyright.

Doherty, P.J. (2006) Physical activity and exercise for patients with implantable cardioverter defibrillators. *British Journal of Cardiac Nursing*, 1, 327–31.

Duncan, G.E., Anton, S.D., Sydeman, Y.S.J., *et al*. (2005) Prescribing exercise at varied levels of intensity and frequency: a randomized trial. *Archives of Internal Medicine*, 165, 2362–9.

Durstine, J.L., Davis, P.G. (2001) Specificity of exercise training and testing. In: *ACSM's Resource Manual for Guidelines for Exercise Testing and Prescription*. Philadelphia, PA: Lippincott Williams & Wilkins, pp. 484–91.

Driving and Vehicle Licensing Agency (DVLA) – At a Glance (DVLA) (2001). Available http://www.dvla.gov.uk/at_a_glance/(accessesd 18 November 2001).

Exner, D.V., Pinski, S.L., Wyse, D.G., *et al*. (2001) Electrical storm presages nonsudden death: The antiarrhythmics versus implantable defibrillators (AVID) trial. *Circulation*, 103, 2066–71.

Fitchet, A., Doherty, P.J., Bundy, C., *et al*. (2003) Comprehensive cardiac rehabilitation programme for implantable cardioverter-defibrillator patients: a randomised controlled trial. *Heart*, 89, 155–60.

Fleg, J.L., Pina, I.L., Balady, G.J., *et al*. (2000) Assessment of functional capacity in clinical and research applications: an advisory from the Committee on Exercise, Rehabilitation, and Prevention, Council on Clinical Cardiology, American Heart Association. *Circulation*, 102, 1591–7.

Fletcher, G.F., Balady, G.J., Amsterdam, E.A., *et al*. (2001) Exercise standards for testing and training: a statement for healthcare professionals from the American Heart Association. *Circulation*, 104, 1694–740.

Frizelle, D.J., Lewin, R.J., Kaye, G., *et al*. (2004) Cognitive–behavioural rehabilitation programme for patients with an implanted cardioverter defibrillator: a pilot study. *British Journal Health Psychology*, 9, 381–92.

Gibbons, R.J., Balady, G.J., Beasley, J.W., *et al*. (1997) American Cardiac College/American Heart Association (ACC/AHA) Guidelines for Exercise Testing. A report of the American College of Cardiology/American Heart Association Task Force on Practice Guidelines (Committee on Exercise Testing). *Journal of the American College of Cardiology*, 30, 260–311.

Gibbons, R.J., Balady, G.J., Brickner, J.T., *et al*. (2002) American Cardiac College/American Heart Association (ACC/AHA) 2002 Guideline update for exercise testing: summary article. A report of the American College of Cardiology/American Heart Association Task Force on Practice Guidelines (Committee to Update the 1997 Exercise Testing Guidelines). *Journal of the American College of Cardiology*, 40, 1531–40.

Hallstrom, A.P., Mcanulty, J.H., Wilkoff, B.L., *et al*. (2001) Patients at lower risk of arrhythmia recurrence: a subgroup in whom implantable defibrillators may not offer benefit. Antiarrhythmics Versus Implantable Defibrillator (AVID) Trial Investigators. *Journal of the American College of Cardiology*, 37, 1093–9.

Heyward, V. (2002) *Advanced Fitness Assessment and Exercise Prescription*, 4h edn. Champaign, IL: Human Kinetics.

Lampman, R.M., Knight, B.P. (2000) Prescribing exercise training for patients with defibrillators. *American Journal of Physical Medicine and Rehabilitation*, 79, 292–7.

Latham, N., Anderson, C., Bennett, D., *et al.* (2003) Progressive resistance strength training for physical disability in older people. *Cochrane Database of Systematic Reviews*, Issue 2. Art No.: CD002759. DOI: 10.1002/14651858.CD002759.

Lee, I.M., Sesso, H.D., Oguma, Y., *et al.* (2003) Relative intensity of physical activity and risk of coronary heart disease. *Circulation*, 107, 1110–16.

Lewin, R.J., Frizelle, D.J., Kaye, G.C. (2001) A rehabilitative approach to patients with internal cardioverter-defibrillators. *Heart*, 85, 371–2.

Luthje, L., Vollmann, D., Rosenfeld, M., *et al.* (2005) Electrogram configuration and detection of supraventricular tachycardias by a morphology discrimination algorithm in single chamber ICDs. *Pacing and Clinical Electrophysiology*, 28, 555–60.

Macauley, D. (1999) *Benifits and Hazards of Exercise*. London: BMJ Publication Group.

Malfatto, G., Facchini, M., Bragato, R., *et al.* (1996) Short and long term effects of exercise training on the tonic autonomic modulation of heart rate variability after myocardial infarction. *European Heart Journal*, 17, 532–8.

Maron, B.J., Shen, W.K., Link, M.S., *et al.* (2000) Efficacy of implantable cardioverter-defibrillators for the prevention of sudden death in patients with hypertrophic cardiomyopathy. *New England Journal of Medicine*, 342, 365–73.

Mayordomo, J., Batalla, A. (2002) Characteristics of patients with ventricular arrhythmias induced with exercise testing. *International Journal of Cardiology*, 83, 299–300.

McArdle, K., Katch, F., Katch, V. (2001) *Exercise Physiology*. Baltimore, MD: Lippincott Williams & Walkins.

McCafferty, W.B., Hovarth, S.M. (1977) Specificity of exercise and specificity of training: A subcellular review. *Research Quarterly*, 48, 358–71.

Moss, A.J., Hall, W.J., Cannom, D.S., *et al.* (1996) Improved survival with an implanted defibrillator in patients with coronary disease at high risk for ventricular arrhythmia. Multicenter Automatic Defibrillator Implantation Trial Investigators. *New England Journal of Medicine*, 335, 1933–40.

Myers, J., Tan, S.Y., Abella, J., *et al.* (2007) Comparison of the chronotropic response to exercise and heart rate recovery in predicting cardiovascular mortality. *European Journal of Cardiovascular Prevention and Rehabilitation*, 14, 215–21.

Namerow, P.B., Firth, B.R., Heywood, G.M., *et al.* (1999) Quality-of-life six months after CABG surgery in patients randomized to ICD versus no ICD therapy: findings from the CABG Patch Trial. *Pacing and Clinical Electrophysiology*, 22, 1305–13.

National Institute of Clinical Excellence (NICE) (2000) *Guidance on the Use of Implantable Cardioverter Defibrillators for Arrhythmias*. London: National Institute for Health and Clinical Excellence, Crown copyright.

National Institute of Clinical Excellence (NICE) (2007) *Implantable Cardioverter Defibrillators for Arrhythmias: Review of Technology Appraisal 11*. London: National Institute for Health and Clinical Excellence, Crown copyright.

Parkes, J., Bryant, J., Milne, R. (2000) Implantable cardioverter defibrillators: arrhythmias. A rapid and systematic review. *Health Technology Assessment*, 4, 1–69.

Pashkow, F.J., Schweikert, R.A., Wilkoff, B.L. (1997) Exercise testing and training in patients with malignant arrhythmias. *Exercise and Sports Science Review*, 25, 235–69.

Pigozzi, F., Alabiso, A., Parisi, A., *et al*. (2004) Vigorous exercise training is not associated with prevalence of ventricular arrhythmias in elderly athletes. *The Journal of Sports Medicine and Physical Fitness*, 44, 92–7.

Pina, I.L., Apstein, C.S., Balady, G.J., *et al*. (2003) Exercise and heart failure: a statement from the American Heart Association Committee on exercise, rehabilitation, and prevention. *Circulation*, 107, 1210–25.

Pinski, S.L., Fahy, G.J. (1995) The proarrhythmic potential of implantable cardioverter-defibrillators. *Circulation*, 92, 1651–64.

Raviele, A., Bongiorni, M.G., Brignole, M., *et al*. (1999) Which strategy is 'best' after myocardial infarction? The Beta-blocker strategy plus implantable cardioverter defibrillator trial: rationale and study design. *American Journal of Cardiology*, 83, 104D–11D.

Rees, K., Taylor, R.S., Singh, S., *et al*. (2004) Exercise based rehabilitation for heart failure. *Cochrane Database Systematic Review*, CD003331.

Richardson, R.S. (2000) What governs skeletal muscle VO_2max? New evidence. *Medicine and Science in Sports and Exercise*, 32, 100–107.

Richardson, R.S., Harms, C.A., Grassi, B., *et al*. (2000) Skeletal muscle: master or slave of the cardiovascular system? *Medicine and Science in Sports and Exercise*, 32, 89–93.

Saltin, B., Nazar, K., Costill, D.L., *et al*. (1976) The nature of the training response: peripheral and central adaptations of one-legged exercise. *Acta Physiologica Scandinavica*, 96, 289–305.

Sears, S.F., Jr, Conti, J.B., Curtis, A.B., *et al*. (1999) Affective distress and implantable cardioverter defibrillators: cases for psychological and behavioural interventions. *Pacing and Clinical Electrophysiology*, 22, 1831–4.

Sears, S.F., Jr, Rauch, S., Handberg, E., *et al*. (2001) Fear of exertion following ICD storm: considering ICD shock and learning history. *Journal of Cardiopulmonary Rehabilitation*, 21, 47–9.

Siebels, J., Kuck, K.H. (1994) Implantable cardioverter defibrillator compared with antiarrhythmic drug treatment in cardiac arrest survivors (the Cardiac Arrest Study Hamburg). *American Heart Journal*, 127, 1139–44.

Singer, I. (1994) AVID necessity. *Pacing and Clinical Electrophysiology*, 17, 260–2; author reply 262–6.

Smart, N., Marwick, T.H. (2004) Exercise training for patients with heart failure: a systematic review of factors that improve mortality and morbidity. *American Journal of Medicine*, 116, 693–706.

Sotile, W.M., and Sears, S.F. (1999) *You Can Make a Difference: Brief Psychosocial Interventions for ICD Patients and Their Families*. Minneapolis, MN: Medtronic Inc.

Thompson, P.D., Franklin, B.A., Balady, G.J., *et al*. (2007) Exercise and acute cardiovascular events placing the risks into perspective: a scientific statement from the American Heart Association Council on Nutrition, Physical Activity, and Metabolism and the Council on Clinical Cardiology. *Circulation*, 115, 2358–68.

Thow, M.K. (ed) (2006). *Exercise Leadership in Cardiac Rehabilitation – An Evidence-based Approach*. West Sussex: Wiley and Sons.

Toner, M.M., Glickman, E.L., Mcardle, W.D. (1990) Cardiovascular adjustments to exercise distributed between the upper and lower body. *Medicine and Science in Sports and Exercise*, 22, 773–8.

Vanhees, L., Kornaat, M., Defoor, J., *et al.* (2004) Effect of exercise training in patients with an implantable cardioverter defibrillator. *European Heart Journal*, 25(13), 1120–26.

Vanhees, L., Schepers, D., Heidbuchel, H., *et al.* (2001) Exercise performance and training in patients with implantable cardioverter-defibrillators and coronary heart disease. *American Journal of Cardiology*, 87(7), 12–15.

Vincent, K.R., Vincent, H.K., Braith, R.W., *et al.* (2003) Strength training and hemodynamic responses to exercise. *American Journal of Geriatric Cardiology*, 12, 97–106.

Wilkoff, B.L. (2006) Pacemaker and ICD malfunction – an incomplete picture. *Journal of the American Medical Association*, 295, 1944–6.

Wilkoff, B.L., Stern, R., Williamson, B., *et al.* (2006) Design of the primary prevention parameters evaluation (PREPARE) trial of implantable cardioverter defibrillators to reduce patient morbidity [NCT00279279]. *Trials*, 7, 18.

Williams, S.G., Cooke, G.A., Wright, D.J., *et al.* (2001) Peak exercise cardiac power output; a direct indicator of cardiac function strongly predictive of prognosis in chronic heart failure. *European Heart Journal*, 22, 1496–503.

5 Heart Transplants

Sue Dennell

Chapter outline

This chapter outlines the indications of heart transplant (HT) and the benefits of exercise for HT, and describes management through physical activity. In addition, guidelines on exercise prescription and monitoring are reviewed. This group of patients provides exercise professionals with considerable challenges due to the denervation of the heart. In addition, controlling rejection of the donor heart by immunosuppressive medications poses further problems for the patient and for exercise professionals. The emphasis of the chapter is on developing safe and practical advice that clinicians and patients can use in decision-making about physical activity and exercise while considering the added problems for HT recipients.

Overview of pathophysiology

Since the first human HT in 1968 in Cape Town, South Africa, where survival of the recipient lasted only days, we now see HT surgery as much more successful, relatively common and performed across the world. Higher survival rates amongst HT recipients have given rise to a larger number of potential candidates for cardiac rehabilitation (CR). In addition, as HT surgery is carried out at a very few select centres of excellence, the patients will be referred to their local CR centres, and subsequently into the community for phase IV, CR exercise professionals will require a sound knowledge of the specific needs of the HT participant. The number of transplants is increasing, with 156 HTs carried out in the UK between January 2006 and December 2006 (United Kingdom Transplant Support Service Authority (UKTSSA), 2007). In 2003 there had been more than 61 000 HTs worldwide, thus not a small number of people receiving this life-saving surgery (Hertz *et al.*, 2002). Due to much improved donor to recipient tissue matching, superior surgical skills and immunosuppressive medications, there is improvement in survival (Hertz *et al.*, 2002). One-year survival of HT recipients in the UK is now in excess of 80% and 5-year survival in excess of 65%. Survival figures for the US show 1-year survival being 86% and their 3-year survival being 80% (American College of Sports

Medicine (ACSM), 2006). Compared to other CR groups the age of recipients of HT is in the younger age groups, with 71% aged between 18 and 59 years. It is well documented that HT recipients have low levels of exercise tolerance. This exercise intolerance for this group is a mixture of factors, including cardiac, neurohormonal, vascular, skeletal muscle and respiratory. In addition, severe deconditioning of the subjects frequently follows on post-transplant from the preoperative period of ill health. Studies have shown that habitual exercise training can improve exercise capacity, muscle mass, muscle strength, bone density and quality of life for this cardiac group (Braith *et al.*, 1992; Haykowsky *et al.*, 2003; Kavanagh *et al.*, 1988; Kobashigawa, 1999; Marconi and Marzorati, 2003). Furthermore, as many of the effects of the immunosuppressive lifetime medications required to prevent rejection by these patients have arteriosclerotic effects, CR is even more important for this group (ACSM, 2006). In addition, there are significant psychosocial benefits for HT subjects who participate in regular exercise.

Indications for heart transplant

Strict criteria are applied to the selection of candidates for transplant because of the scarcity of donor organs in the UK. Although there is no age limit, with all biologically fit candidates being considered for transplant, there is an increase in possible comorbidity with increasing age that may adversely affect the patient's outcome. For most patients, if they do not receive a transplant their life expectancy is often limited to 12–24 months. For a successful outcome recipients should be well enough to withstand the surgery, the stresses of postoperative recovery and immunosuppressive medication therapy, and should have the potential for good physical function. Most patients presenting for assessment of cardiac transplant have severe ventricular dysfunction, with classes III–IV heart failure on the New York Heart Association Scale (see Table 3.1) and poor quality of life, despite maximal medical therapy, including previous cardiac resynchronisation therapy. Low peak VO_2 of less than 14 mL/kg/min, or if on β-blocker therapy, less than 12 mL/kg/min, has been shown to correlate with other markers of unfavourable disease severity. Other markers including ejection fraction, pulmonary capillary wedge pressure, type of heart failure and cardiac index are used as selection indicators for potential transplant recipients (Mancini *et al.*, 1991; Mudge *et al.*, 1993; Myers *et al.*, 1998; UKTSSA, 2007).

The types of patients who receive transplant are varied, and within the last decade the reasons for transplant have remained much the same (Taylor *et al.*, 2005). The largest group consists of those with poor left ventricular function, secondary to coronary artery disease. Cardiomyopathies of various aetiologies comprise the second-largest group. Transplant is also carried out for congenital heart disease, valvular disease, adult congenital heart disease or severe intractable angina that is not amenable to other therapies and refractory ventricular dysrhythmias.

Criteria for possible transplant candidates

Candidates for transplant should not have any serious systemic disease or other medical condition that may affect the outcome of transplant. The candidate should have a body mass index of $<30 \, kg/m^2$. They must have a good understanding of the procedure, with the possible limitations of the procedure and possible adverse effects of medical therapy. The candidate should be counselled on the long-term compliance required with drug therapy. In addition, the recipient will require many clinic attendances post-procedure. To optimise the outcome they should have a strong social and family support network. Finally, they should be free from substance, nicotine or alcohol abuse prior to their surgery.

Rehabilitation of the HT patient begins as soon as the patient is presented for assessment, in order to maintain the patient in the best possible condition prior to surgery, in preparation for the period of postoperative recovery. Optimal medical therapy to control heart failure symptoms allows all ambulatory patients to exercise. Some may attend chronic heart failure rehabilitation session, but this is not yet available in all areas. For other patients, daily walks or an exercise regime of around 15 exercises, each carried out for a minute at home, can help to maintain leg strength, particularly, increasing exercise capability. During each minute of exercise, pace and number of repetitions can be altered to accommodate symptoms of breathlessness and muscle fatigue. Examples of exercises used are alternating flexion through elevation of the arms, straight leg lifts, half squats, alternate hip abduction, marching on the spot and hip flexion/extension.

For the same ejection fraction, exercise tolerance between patients may vary widely. The reasons for this variation are not only haemodynamic dysfunction caused by their heart disease. Factors such as muscle deconditioning, secondary to bed rest or limited ability to exercise, contribute to ever-decreasing exercise capability. Patients in congestive cardiac failure have disordered muscle metabolism, with abnormally rapid depletion of phosphocreatine and greater intracellular acidosis. This derangement worsens as heart failure advances (Stratton *et al.*, 1994). There is no potential for improvement of cardiac function at this time; any improvement in exercise tolerance comes about through increasing the strength of peripheral skeletal muscle.

Surgery for heart transplant

Anaesthesia, median sternotomy and heart–lung bypass are carried out in a similar way to that for cardiac surgery prior to the transplant procedure. Two alternative techniques for orthotopic transplant are employed: the standard procedure of Lower and Shumway or the bicaval Wythenshawe technique described by the Manchester group in the early nineties (Sarsam *et al.*, 1993).

In the standard procedure the recipient heart is removed by incising the atria, pulmonary artery and aorta. The posterior walls of both atria, including the sinoatrial node, are left intact. Four anastomoses are then carried out: left atrial, right atrial, pulmonary artery and aortic. The P-wave of both the donor and the recipient sinoatrial node may therefore be discernible on the postoperative ECG.

The bicaval Wythenshawe technique has the advantage of maintaining the normal size and shape of the atria, particularly right atrium. The entire right atrium is excised. Anastomoses are then carried out: left atrial, inferior vena cava, superior vena cava, pulmonary artery and aortic. Comparison of the two techniques by various groups demonstrated that the bicaval recipients had a lower right atrial pressure, better atrial contractility, better sinus node competence, with lower likelihood of atrial tachyarrhythmias and less need for pacing, lower incidence and severity of tricuspid valve dysfunction, lower need for diuretic therapy and a shorter hospital stay (el-Gamel *et al.*, 1995; Grant *et al.*, 1995). Although reinnervation of the heart is rare, it is thought to occur more readily in patients with a transplant carried out using the bicaval technique (Bernardi *et al.*, 1998). Improved medium-term survival has also been reported (Aziz *et al.*, 1999). The bicaval Wythenshawe technique has been adopted by many cardiac transplant centres worldwide. Both the standard and the bicaval techniques are orthotopic techniques of transplantation, in which the recipient heart is almost completely replaced by the donor heart. The heterotopic technique of heart transplantation in which the donor heart is anastomosed to the recipient heart 'piggyback' fashion is rarely used now. Exercise therapy is therefore described for orthotopic transplant recipients.

Denervation of cardiac efferent nerves

In cardiac transplant recipients the heart is denervated at operation (Banner *et al.*, 1989). Despite the differences in cardiac dynamics between transplanted and normally innervated individuals, transplanted patients can benefit from exercise training. There is a loss of vagal efferent tone to the sinoatrial node, resulting in a rise of the resting heart rate of approximately 30%. Normal increase in the heart rate through exercise haemorrhage and vasodilatation is attenuated. In addition, there is less reduction of heart rate variability when posture is altered from supine to the standing position, compared with normal individuals who experience an immediate reflex rise in heart rate (Yusuf *et al.*, 1987). Neither does the rate alter in response to the Valsalva manoeuvre (the forced effort of the breath against a closed throat) or carotid sinus massage (Kavanagh, 1996).

Denervation of cardiac afferent nerves

Heart transplantation interrupts key neural and humoral homeostatic mechanisms that adjust sodium and fluid balance. Lack of cardiac afferent information to the hypothalamus and medulla oblongata that normally buffer neuroendocrine activity allows neuroendocrine hyperactivity of the renin–angiotensin–aldosterone system of the kidney. This leads to a lack of response to hypervolemic stimulus, leading to fluid retention and therefore increased circulating blood volume of up to 14%. This may be partly responsible for the incidence of hypertension in HT recipients (Braith *et al.*, 1992; Eisen 2003). Denervation of cardiac afferent information may also cause loss of control of the peripheral vasculature and loss of the sensation of cardiac pain in the presence of cardiac vessel atherosclerosis in the graft (Keteyian *et al.*, 1989). Total denervation of the heart results in little or no change in heart rate when posture is altered from supine to the sitting position.

Implications of denervation on exercise for heart transplant

There is no reflex rise in heart rate through sympathetic stimulation on commencing exercise. There is a loss of vagal tone to the sinoatrial node (Banner *et al.*, 1988; Kavanagh *et al.*, 1988). The resulting resting tachycardia implies a low stroke volume. Therefore, there is potential for a rise in stroke volume of up to 20% because of increased diastolic filling through increased venous return from working muscles and the pulmonary pump of ventilation increasing preload (Frank–Starling mechanism) (Pflugfelder *et al.*, 1987). The Bainbridge reflex, represented by intrinsic stretch of cardioacceleratory fibres in the right atrium, gives a small rise in heart rate early in exercise. As exercise continues, positive chronotropic action of circulating catecholamines increases heart rate, but this is insufficient to increase myocardial contractility to the same degree as sympathetic stimulation (Kavanagh *et al.*, 1988; Robson *et al.*, 1989). Heart rate and blood pressure response to exercise are attenuated because of denervation and cannot therefore be used to determine end points for exercise. Ventilation and oxygen uptake start to increase immediately on exercise, despite a lack of cardiac efferents, demonstrating that ventilation is not causally linked to right ventricular output or work (Banner *et al.*, 1988).

Implications of denervation on ceasing exercise for heart transplant

On ceasing exercise, there will be a slow decline in heart rate because of the absence of vagal activity to put a brake on the sinoatrial node. Slow removal of endogenous catecholamines that have built up in the circulation on exercise will take 10–15 minutes to be removed. Ceasing exercise abruptly following steady intensive exercise where the heart rate has become elevated may therefore cause blood pressure to drop below baseline levels, as venous return from working muscle drops but the heart rate remains high. Thus, longer cool-down periods will be required as recovery takes longer (ACSM, 2006).

Activity in phase I cardiac rehabilitation for heart transplant

Exercise rehabilitation can commence when the patient is recovering from the transplant procedure. There may be some variation between transplant units, but the inpatient stay for an uncomplicated patient will be around 3 weeks. Exercise will commence as soon as the patient is extubated and most of the intensive monitoring has ceased. Beginning with active leg exercises on the bed, the patient will rapidly progress to standing exercises and walking, and until around the fourth or fifth day they will be walking freely around the ward and beginning to incorporate stair climbing. The patient will start to exercise in the physiotherapy from the time of their first endomyocardial biopsy at around 7 days postoperatively, provided that there is little or no rejection. Cycle ergometry may be introduced at this point with no resistance, step-ups on a 6-inch step, treadmill walking at a slow pace, gradually increasing duration. Intensity of exercise may be set by not allowing oxygen saturation to fall below 92%, with respiratory rate not rising above 30 breaths/min. Use of the rate of perceived exertion (RPE) on the Borg 6–20 scale can be commenced, encouraging patients to work at levels 11–13 (fairly light to somewhat hard) (Borg, 1998). In addition, they should use muscle fatigue and shortness of breath to further determine their exercise limits throughout the rehabilitation process. Some lightweight work will be included in the gym session in order to start to build up muscle strength in the legs, keeping the weight low and the repetitions high.

Strenuous arm exercises are avoided at this time in order to allow the sternum to heal. Only free arm movements and very lightweights in the order of 0.5 kg are used during exercise. Following cardiac surgery, healing usually takes place over approximately 6 weeks. As transplanted patients receive steroid medication, this may delay bony union, so that more strenuous arm exercises are added from 8 weeks onwards, around the time that they may commence outpatient phase III rehabilitation in their local area. (Guidelines for resumption of physical activity are shown in Table 5.1; Ainsworth *et al.*, 2002.) These guidelines provide suggestions of progression of exercise and activity for HT recipients. These guidelines should be used in conjunction with the individuals' health status, cardiovascular risk factor profile, medications, exercise behaviour, patients' personal goals and their exercise preferences (ACSM, 2006).

Table 5.1 Guidelines for activity during recovery and rehabilitation following transplant.

Time	Energy expenditure	Activities of daily living	Occupational activity	Exercise
Up to 6 weeks postoperatively	Very light <3 METs <10 mL/kg/min	Washing, shaving, dressing; washing dishes; food preparation; ironing small items; stair climbing	Desk work – sedentary, clerical activities	Gentle walking <2 miles/hour; static cycle, no resistance; very light calisthenics (aerobic movements akin to warm-up activity)
At 6 weeks postoperatively	Light 3–5 METs 11–18 mL/kg/min	Cleaning windows; mopping; light vacuuming; raking leaves; light weeding; powered lawn mowing; carrying objects 7–11 kg; driving short distances	Stocking shelves; light welding, carpentry, machine assembly; light electrical work	Brisker walking (3–4 miles/hour); level cycling outdoors (6–8 miles/hour); light aerobics with some light-resistance work; social badminton; bowling
At 8 weeks postoperatively	Moderate 5–7 METs 18–25 mL/kg/min	Easy garden digging and planting; hanging out heavy wet washing; changing bed linen; carrying objects 11–22 kg; using crutches	Joinery, shovelling light loads; using heavier tools; light ladder work; masonry	Walking (4.5–5.0 miles/hour); cycling (9–10 miles/hour or 100–150 W); aerobic activities and moderate-resistance work; dancing; fishing; golf
At 12 weeks postoperatively	Heavy 7–9 METs 25–32 mL/kg/min	Heavier shovelling, sawing wood; paper hanging; carrying objects 22–35 kg	Exterior joinery, digging ditches, hay baling; tree surgery; using heavy tools	Football; swimming; cycling uphill or 12–13 miles/hour; jogging 6 miles/hour; aerobics rigorous effort; circuit training; step aerobics 6- to 8-inch steps
At 16 weeks postoperatively	Very heavy >9 METs >32 mL/kg/min	Carrying loads upstairs	Heavy labour	Running briskly (it is not recommended to take up long-distance jogging/running as a new pastime); cycling 14.0–15.9 miles/hour; scuba diving; rock climbing

Ainsworth *et al.* (2002).

Activity in phase II cardiac rehabilitation for heart transplant

Between discharge and commencement of a supervised rehabilitation pro-gramme, the patient may be discharged with a daily walking regime, whereby they gradually increase their distance by 100 yards each day, starting with a distance that they have managed easily in hospital. They should maintain a walking pace up to an RPE of 13. As a simple guide they should have enough breath to walk and talk at the same time. Within these restrictions they should gradually be able to increase the speed and gradient of their walking as their fitness and confidence increase. All CR patient groups should increase their activity by incorporating an active lifestyle. This encourages an increase in daily activity where activity is accumulated over a day (ACSM, 2006). The message behind this encour-ages moderate-intensity exercise, accumulating 30 minutes or more per day on most, preferably all, days of the week (Pate *et al.*, 1995). The activity can be accumulated in multiple small 'bouts' of activity, for example three 10-minute bouts of walking.

This stage encourages active living, using the stairs instead of the es-calator, walking the children to school instead of driving, etc. Despite the intensity being too low to gain significant improvements in aerobic fit-ness, ACSM (2006) has shown that activity at this lower intensity will offer substantial benefits across a broad range of health outcomes.

There is not an automatic improvement in exercise ability post-transplant, and patients will benefit greatly from a structured exercise programme (Marconi and Marzorati, 2003). Comparison of early post-transplant patients in a supervised 6-month exercise programme with a group receiving unstructured home therapy showed that the super-vised group had an increase in peak oxygen consumption and workload and greater reduction in ventilatory equivalent for carbon dioxide. Re-jection episodes, antihypertensive medications, infections, prednisolone dose and body weight did not differ significantly between the two groups (Kobashigawa, 1999).

Assessment of heart transplant patients prior to phase III

Prior to phase III, assessment should begin with knowledge of the patient's latest cardiac biopsy result, as rejection can impair exercise performance. If at any time there is a sign of rejection, the phase III programme should be ceased until reversal of rejection. An exercise test prior to commencing an exercise programme is of value, despite the attenuated heart rate and blood pressure response, in order to determine exercise intensity and pro-vide baseline measurements for future comparison. Aerobic test protocols should allow time for an appropriate increase in heart rate and oxygen consumption at each workload. Exercise testing can be carried out on a cycle ergometer ramp protocol of 10–15 W/min or a treadmill, but performance is usually lower (6–11%) on a cycle ergometer than on a treadmill. Exercise protocols that last approximately 10–14 minutes, consisting of 3- to 5-minute stages with one metabolic equivalent (MET) increments at each stage, allow the denervated heart to respond to the increasing workload. A suitable protocol for debilitated individuals is the Naughton, in which lower speeds are used than in a full Bruce protocol, with a one MET increase per stage. A modified Bruce may also be used. The 6-minute walk test is also suggested by the ACSM (2003) to measure endurance. The 6-minute test may have some benefits as little or no equipment is required to carry it out. A drawback of the 6-minute test is the difficulty in monitoring the patients during the test and patients not able to pace themselves.

Ideally a treadmill test should be carried out with collection of expired gases to determine maximal effort. This is shown by reaching an oxygen plateau, a failure of oxygen intake to rise despite an increase in workload. The measurement of blood lactate will allow determination of the ventilatory threshold, the level of exertion at which there is a disproportionate rise in blood lactate. Exercise beyond this point becomes increasingly anaerobic. This ventilatory threshold is the level of exercise intensity preferred for cardiac patients and other debilitated patients. It occurs at an oxygen intake of 50–65% of VO_2max in normal and HT patients (Kavanagh, 1996). If it is not possible to carry out expired gas analysis, maximal exertion can be determined from the patients.

If it is not possible to carry out expired gas analysis, maximal exertion can be determined from the patient's level of work when they reach the RPE of 19–20 on the Borg scale which is 'very very hard' on the scale (Borg, 1998). Ventilatory threshold can be decided from the point in the test where the RPE was rated at 12–14 (somewhat hard). This level of exercise intensity can then be translated in terms of exercise pace during CR sessions of resistance exercise (RE), aerobic exercise, treadmill walking/jogging and cycle ergometer power output. The following should be noted during an exercise test: resting sinus tachycardia, blood pressure, delayed heart rate and blood pressure response, two separate P-waves on the ECG (if the patient has had the standard rather than the bicaval procedure) and delayed recovery of the heart rate to pre-exercise levels. ECG, blood pressure and RPE should be noted at each stage during the exercise test. The ACSM (2003) suggests that RPE is a better estimate of exercise intensity due to the delayed/blunting heart response. During the first year after transplant whilst a patient's physical capabilities improve rapidly, exercise testing should be carried out at regular intervals in order to ensure that the exercise training intensity remains optimal.

Phase III exercise prescription for heart transplant

Exercise prescription should be part of a holistic plan that includes diet, weight control, drug therapy, with advice on medication effects and side effects, and ongoing patient education. Exercise rehabilitation in phase III can commence as early as 8 weeks postoperatively, once the sternum has healed. Goals are to improve health, reduce the risk and severity of cardiovascular disease, improve physical capacity in terms of strength and endurance and ensure safety, preventing injury and not aggravating any chronic conditions.

Exercise training should be matched to specific goals and should include aerobic training, skeletal muscle strengthening, flexibility, balance and skill improvements. The extent to which improvement takes place is related to the duration, mode, intensity and frequency of training. As with other exercise prescription the consensus suggests that the frequency, intensity, timing and type of exercise are the primary determinants of the exercise training effect (ACSM, 2006). If correct exercise prescription is carried out, improvements can be made not only to cardiorespiratory fitness of HT subjects but also to general health, disease prevention and psychosocial well-being (Karapolat *et al.*, 2007; Scottish Intercollegiate Guidelines Network (SIGN), 2002).

To achieve these improvements any exercise programme must work the body systems harder than it is normally accustomed to. This process is known as overload and can be applied to any aspect of exercise, including cardiovascular fitness, strength and flexibility training (ACSM, 2006). The body responds to the specific exercise stimulus by adapting to the increased exercise load. For example an individual who is sedentary can overload their system by walking at a faster pace than normal for an increasingly longer time and more frequently. An individual who has been more active for a period of time will require their activity overload to be set at a higher intensity and/or to work for longer periods to maintain improvement. Gradually, as the individual adjusts to the exercise, future bouts of exercise will need to be increased in order to continue to achieve overload. This process is known as progressive overload, and it should continue until the individual's agreed training CR goals are achieved.

In order to achieve this overload, the exercise professional must consider the FITT(E), where the E stands for enjoyment. This principle describes the relationship between frequency, intensity, time and type of exercise, and it is an essential tool when prescribing effective exercise for any person wishing to improve health-related fitness. Exercise prescription must be individualised to increase the likelihood of enjoyment (E). Enjoyment of exercise has significant implications for adherence to exercise in a CR setting (Thow *et al.*, 2008). Thus, exercise professionals should strive to make the exercise experience an enjoyable and fun one to favourably influence adherence. Table 5.2 summarises exercise prescription for HT recipients.

Table 5.2 Summary of exercise prescription for phase III for heart transplant recipients.

Component of training	Frequency (sessions per week)	Intensity	Duration	Activity
Cardiorespiratory	3–6 days/week and adopt healthy living activity	50–75% VO$_2$peak or HHR RPE 11–12 to 14–15	15–60 minutes Minimum of 16 weeks	Dynamic activity of large muscles, e.g. walk/jog and aerobic circuit
Resistance	3–6 sessions per week	60% one RM	1–3 sets, 12–15 repetitions	Major muscle groups, e.g. free weights and Theraband

HHR, heart rate reserve; RPE, rating of perceived exertion; RM, repetition maximum.

FITTE stands for the following:

F, frequency (number of days per week)
I, intensity (exertion required)
T, time (minutes per day and duration of programme)
T, type (specific mode of activity)
E, enjoyment (pleasurable experience of the participant)

Due to the altered heart rate responses and extended recovery time, a longer warm-up and cool-down may be required for HT patients (ACSM, 2006). In a normal CR warm-up, a period of 15 minutes used for HT up to 20 minutes may be necessary. The exercise professional will need to assess each individual and take into consideration their exercise capacity and the need to extend or not the warm-up and cool-down sections of the structured exercise session.

The frequency of training sessions should be at least three up to six times a week (ACSM, 2006), depending on the initial fitness and desired goals of the individual. If supervised exercise cannot be provided at this frequency, the patient can carry out the activities at home for two to three sessions a week, once they have been educated in exercise content, self-monitoring and the use of RPE. As with other CR groups the exercise professional should provide the HT subject with an individualised home exercise programme to increase their exposure to their training dose. There is some evidence that for the HT CR patients, a well-structured, supportive, hospital-based phase III CR compared to a similar home programme is the best method of delivery to improve post-surgical exercise capacity measured by VO$_2$max and quality of life measured by the Short Form 36 and Beck Depression Inventory (Karapolat *et al.*, 2007).

Exercise intensity remains the most critical, yet the most difficult, component of the exercise prescription to establish. A MET level at or slightly below ventilatory threshold (where the patient starts to increase the rate and depth of breathing), or an RPE of between 11–12 and 14–15, or a VO_2peak between 50 and 75%, may be used to establish the initial level of exercise intensity (ACSM, 2006; Badenhop, 1995; Kavanagh, 1996). Using RPE, however, it has been found that during exercise testing males and females varied in perception over two different exercise protocols. There were significant differences in the rating of RPE at 40, 60 and 80% of maximum heart rate reserve between the two protocols and that men rated each of the RPE intensities significantly higher than women. These perceptual differences between the protocols could not be accounted for by physiological measures assessed within this study. Large interindividual variations of RPE limit the value of perceived exertion in exercise prescription. Ratings may be more suited to fine-tuning fixed-distance/fixed-speed exercise prescriptions during rehabilitation following transplant (Shephard *et al.*, 1996; Whaley *et al.*, 1997).

Each session should last 15–60 minutes, depending on the capabilities of the patient (ACSM, 2006). Initially, a patient may have reached the limits of endurance by completing a warm-up session, and further activity will have to be incorporated gradually. The exercise professional will need to be aware of these patients with the initial low levels of function. The duration of the programme should be more than 16 weeks in order to see an increase in exercise tolerance and the added benefits of habitual exercise (Keteyian *et al.*, 1989). As many CR programmes in the UK are 8–12 weeks in duration, special provision may have to be made to accommodate transplanted patients in phase IV or HT subjects should remain in phase III for up to 4 months.

The type or mode of training should include a warm-up of exercises consisting of repetitive low-level aerobic movements and stretching of major muscle groups prior to the main overload part of the programme in order to allow a rise in circulating catecholamine levels and therefore heart rate. Any suitable rhythmic dynamic exercise of cardiovascular exercise, involving the main large muscle groups of the upper and lower body, should be used to achieve cardiovascular training effects. The modes of training may vary from programme to programme due to availability of equipment and facilities, but may include aerobic circuit training, walking, jogging, cycle ergometry, rowing, step-ups, treadmill walking/jogging and arm ergometry (see Figure 5.1). The mode of training used should incorporate the needs and goals of the patient.

In the cool-down section there should be a focus on increasing flexibility or range of motion (ROM). These stretches are also called developmental stretches where the aim of the stretching is to increase range of movement over time. These exercises are important for all CR groups but with all major joints should be targeted to improve body function (ACSM, 2003). ROM exercises are particularly important for HT recipients who have a sternotomy; due to post-surgical sternal pain they may adopt poor posture. The aim of cool-down ROM stretching is to maintain range of movement

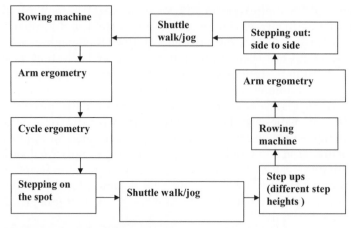

Figure 5.1 CR exercise circuit content example.

and, if required, to improve flexibility of specific muscles (ACSM, 2006). Stretching and increasing ROM is particularly important to reduce adaptive shortening of the pectoral muscles and to maintain thoracic/upper body mobility.

Developmental stretches should be held for between 15 and 30 seconds with four repetitions of each muscle group (ACSM, 2006). The patients should be encouraged to breathe normally, ease into the stretch and not to bounce. The stretch should be carried out in a slow, controlled way. The stretch should be taken to a point of slight discomfort, but not pain. The exercise professional and assistants should be observing participants' performance for position and quality of the exercise and should correct poor technique.

Resistance exercise

Progressive RE training has potential to increase muscle strength and increase bone density (Braith *et al.*, 1993b, 1998; Haykowsky *et al.*, 2003). In addition, resistance training performed for up to 6 months has been found to prevent skeletal muscle loss and increase the patient's fat-free mass to pre-surgery levels (ACSM, 2006). RE incorporates all types of strength and weight trainings and will lead to improvements in both muscle strength and endurance. REs have many proven health benefits, including increases in lean muscular mass, and it has been shown to complement aerobic exercise in the maintenance of basal metabolic rate, important for weight management. In addition, RE can reduce the risk of falling by improving muscular strength and balance (ACSM, 2006). Favourable effects on bone density are associated with RE (Bjarnason-Wehrens *et al.*, 2004). Resistance training may be incorporated into the exercise programme following the aerobic exercise component and cool-down activities, depending on programme in order to allow a gradual decrease of heart rate and circulating catecholamines. Furthermore, the body core temperature will not have returned to resting; therefore, the muscles and connective tissues are still warm. Resistance activities should be carried out for six to eight major muscle groups at 60% of the 1 repetition maximum for 12–15 repetitions using free weights, fixed weight machines or different resistance of Theraband bands. A useful website resource for Theraband (http://www.therabandacademy.com) provides a database of exercises using different loading of elastic bands and allows one to create a printed handout for the patient similar to Physiotools (2005).

Other considerations for exercise

Much of the training effect occurs through changes to peripheral adaptation (Kavanagh *et al.*, 1988), with 24% attributed to peripheral adaptation and 11% to central changes (Tegtbur *et al.*, 2005). These changes are limited initially by poor musculature, as disuse atrophy and defects of muscle metabolism associated with heart failure may persist from the preoperative period (Banner *et al.*, 1988; Kavanagh, 1996; Lampert, 1996). Isometric exercise can cause a rise in systolic and diastolic blood pressure, resulting from an increase in peripheral resistance, but unlike for normally innervated patients, there is no rise in heart rate or stroke volume (Haskell *et al.*, 1981; Kavanagh *et al.*, 1988).

The coronary arteries are not involved in the transplant procedure, as the aorta is resected above their origin. It should be noted that the age limit of donors has increased in recent years, and therefore the risk of donor coronary heart disease is present. Patients with post-transplant angiographic evidence of coronary disease become a higher risk group for subsequent cardiac events (Uretsky *et al.*, 1992). There is clear evidence of the protective role of the parasympathetic control of the cardiovascular system in normal innervated hearts (Leon, 2000) that is lost owing to cardiac denervation.

Benefits of exercise for heart transplant recipients

Following exercise training there is an increase in aerobic exercise capacity. The increased work capacity in turn enhances the quality of life and increases the sense of well-being (Marconi and Marzorati, 2003). The improvements in aerobic performance in HT recipients seem to rest on the improvements in the peripheral muscles' oxidative capacity and general function (Lampert *et al.*, 1998). Tegtbur *et al.* (2005) carried out a study of 21 HT recipients performing a 1-year aerobic individualised training programme compared to 9 HT controls. The HT subjects had experienced their surgery 5.2 ± 2.1 years previously. They monitored the possible time courses for physical adaptation and concluded that the enhancement in cardiovascular exercise function was 24% attributable to improved skeletal muscle function and 11% to central functioning. Interestingly, the largest increase in cardiovascular functioning occurred within the first 3 months of training. This study indicates that HT subjects have the potential to enhance their physical capacity sometime after surgery. Thus, sustained aerobic training can counteract the effects of immunosuppressive medications sometime after surgery. The decrease in resting heart rate, blood pressure, RPE and rate of ventilation also occurs. Aerobic training in normally innervated subjects would see these effects come about through increased vagal tone (sympathetic nervous system). In the transplanted individual there is no vagal connection to bring this about. It has been shown that the denervated heart develops increased sensitivity to circulating catecholamines. There is also evidence that vigorously trained normal and post-infarct patients develop a significant reduction in effort-induced levels of noradrenalin. This may partly explain the mechanism of these effects of training (Kavanagh, 1988). An accelerated form of coronary atherosclerosis develops over time partly due to medications, a slowly progressive diffuse atherosclerosis of chronic rejection, so that at 5 years post-surgery around 45% of patients have angiographic evidence of disease and at 9.5 years post-surgery this increases to 53% (Taylor *et al.*, 2005). Impaired endothelial function is detectable in HT recipients and is regarded as a risk factor for coronary vasculopathy. Coronary vasodilatation driven by bioavailability of nitric oxide, produced by the activities of endothelial-derived enzyme nitric oxide synthase, is disturbed in persons with coronary disease. This, along with excessive oxidative stress, results in loss of endothelial cells. Aggravation of endothelial dysfunction ensues. This triggers myocardial ischaemia in persons with coronary disease. Regular aerobic activity restores vascular function in those patients who are at considerable risk of developing vascular complications (Schmidt *et al.*, 2002).

Postoperative prednisolone is frequently used as part of the recipient's immunosuppressive regime, leading to or exacerbating osteoporosis and a decrease in lean muscle mass. The duration of training, weight-bearing exercise and the use of an RE component have been shown to counter this problem (Braith *et al.*, 1993b; Haykowsky *et al.*, 2003). The following summarises the benefits of exercise for HT recipients:

1. Increase in lean body mass
2. Reduction in heart rate and blood pressure at rest and given submaximal workload and reduced RPE
3. Increase in peak VO_2, peak power output and ventilatory threshold
4. Improved psychological well-being
5. Improved activities of daily life
6. Assist with return to work

(Marconi and Marzorati, 2003).

Factors affecting exercise performance for heart transplant recipients

Transplanted patients regularly compete in UK, European and World Transplant Games. Other transplant patients will compete in long-distance runs, including half and full marathons. Exercise training is effective in improving exercise tolerance in HT recipients, but not to the same extent as in normally innervated individuals. Central haemodynamic abnormalities limit peripheral adaptations to exercise rehabilitation, reducing these individuals' ability to train. Although the transplant patient may not be able to reach the volume and intensity of other innervated athletes, they may achieve levels of physical performance above that of less fit sedentary individuals. This was found by Rochus *et al.* (2004) when testing athletes prior to the European Heart and Lung Transplant Games. Levels of performances of HT athletes have included running a full marathon (over 26 miles) in less than 6 hours (Kavanagh *et al.*, 1986). It should be noted as did Thow *et al.* (2004) with a post-MI patient group that although some cardiac patients can train and achieve relatively higher than average fitness for age-matched subjects, training at these higher levels is suitable only for a small percentage of any cardiac group. In addition, it will only be a small percentage that will be able to or want to train at these higher intensities.

Peak heart rate reached during exercise is significantly lower than that in normally innervated subjects. There is a lower peak VO_2 and increased CO_2 production, compared with healthy subjects. Decreased peak oxygen consumption may partly be explained by skeletal muscle weakness (Braith *et al.*, 1993a).

There is evidence that patients may regain more or less normal lung volumes, airway function and lung haemodynamics after transplant surgery (Marconi and Marzorati, 2003). In some HT subjects there may be impairment of pulmonary diffusing capacity related to preoperative heart failure. It has been suggested that permanent damage to the alveolar capillary membrane may be a result of the patient having long-standing pre-transplant chronic heart failure (Marconi and Marzorati, 2003). In addition, the pulmonary impairment may be contributed to by the use of cyclosporine (Braith *et al.*, 1996). Heart failure patients presenting for transplant will all have preoperative lung function tests, demonstrating low diffusing capacity. This may mask underlying lung disease, for example chronic obstructive pulmonary disease and emphysema. Other factors include a low-tidal-volume response to exercise, compared with normal individuals secondary to mechanical factors such as respiratory muscle weakness, hypoperfusion, long-term deconditioning and long-term use of corticosteroids (Brubaker *et al.*, 1997). Transplant patients with decreased diffusion capacity have a lower exercise tolerance than transplant patients with a normal diffusing capacity. However, because of the lack of exercise-induced hypoxaemia, diffusion abnormalities are not the main limiting factor for low exercise tolerance in the group of patients with low diffusing capacity (Ville *et al.*, 1998). There is decreased oxygen delivery to peripheral working skeletal muscles (Kavanagh, 1996). Ventricular volumes are reduced, but filling pressures are normal, indicating diastolic dysfunction. Possible mechanisms include a mismatch between the donor heart size and the recipient body size, the number of rejections, elevated blood pressure and myocardial ischaemia from the cardiac allograft vasculopathy. In addition, some dysfunction is found in the myocardium in brain-dead donors (Marconi and Marzorati, 2003).

Skeletal muscle limitations may be as a result of the damage due to heart failure pre-transplant. This has been well demonstrated in heart failure patients where abnormalities of muscle structure and metabolic response to exercise are seen. This has been attributed to reduced oxygen extraction capabilities, vascular insufficiency and reduced oxygen supply and/or metabolic flaws within the muscle (Mancini *et al.*, 1992). (See Chapter 3 for more on heart failure.)

Other outcome measures for heart transplant patients

Repeating the exercise test at regular intervals to ensure optimal exercise intensity also gives the opportunity to record improvements in exercise performance. Furthermore, as with all outcome measures for patients, regular feedback on change and improvements can act as a great incentive and motivation. Regular feedback, in turn, can help with adherence to exercise regimes. Aerobic, endurance and strength will be those used in phase III (see pp. 143–144). Handgrip dynamometry correlates well with lean muscle mass and may be repeated easily as a measure of improvement to muscle strength. Electrical impedance monitors, as well as indicating increased muscle mass, will also indicate measure levels of body fat. Spirometry values, peak flow, FEV1 (forced expiratory volume in 1 second) and FVC (forced vital capacity) can easily be reproduced and will demonstrate improving lung function following rehabilitation. In addition, monitoring and early detection of deteriorating pulmonary function is important. As with other respiratory groups such as asthma adherence to home spirometry measurement can be low. HT recipients' adherence was improved by 30% when they were given structured ongoing education on use of spirometry (De Geest *et al.*, 2005).

Psychological outcomes for heart transplant recipients
Psychological problems have been identified in HT recipients primarily due to the lifetime multifaceted therapeutic regimen required to have optimal benefits of HT. The psychological impact includes higher anger, hostility and anxiety. In addition, lower motivation and self-efficacy are common in HT patients (De Geest *et al.*, 2005). Levels of anxiety and depression are found in approximately 50% of patients prior to transplant, with many experiencing ongoing psychiatric and psychological problems

(Ulubay *et al.*, 2007). The experience of preoperative and postoperative HT recipients is psychologically demanding for both patients and families, and the psychological status post-transplant has a considerable impact on compliance with medical management and exercise participation. As the emotional and psychological status is a significant factor, it is important that regular monitoring and measuring of HT recipients' psychological status is advised. HT patients' psychological status can be assessed using simple outcome measures, including the Hospital Anxiety and Depression Scale (SIGN, 2002), Beck Depression Inventory and the State–Trait Anxiety Inventory (Karpolat *et al.*, 2007). If HT patients engage in exercise-based CR, they often experience improvements in psychological status, confidence and well-being. Thus behaviour change strategies to improve exercise uptake and adherence will be imperative for this group.

Medication for heart transplant recipients

Antirejection therapy will continue for lifetime following transplantation. Rejection may be cellular or humoral. The primary mediator of cellular rejection is the activated T-lymphocyte (T cell), although humoral B cells contribute. Acute cellular rejection can occur at any time, but it is most common in the first 3–6 months after transplant. Acute humoral rejection (also called vascular rejection) is much less common (around 7% of patients) and occurs days to weeks after HT and is initiated by antibodies rather than T cells and is directed against donor HLA or endothelial cell antigens. As in cellular rejection, this is treated with alterations in medication to intensify immunosuppression, but also with medication directed specifically at regulating antibody production or removing antibody, such as cyclophosphamide immunoglobulin or plasmapheresis. Endothelial injury and dysfunction are associated with chronic rejection, so humoral (vascular) rejection is associated with increased risk of chronic rejection (Pope, 1980).

Acute cellular rejection occurs after the first 6 months. This usually happens in patients who have had significant rejection early after transplant, a recent reduction in immunosuppressive therapy, an infection, or are non-compliant with medication. Non-compliance may result in rapid onset of serious rejection, and the consequent damage to the graft may not be reversible. Introduction of the drug cyclosporine A in the late 1970s to early 1980s revolutionised heart transplantation, leading to immediate and dramatic improvement in graft and patient survival rates. Cyclosporine may still be used in combination with other drugs to target several steps in T-cell activation, allowing lower doses of each individual drug to minimise side effects. Combination therapy comprises three basic medication groups, the foundation of immunosuppressive therapy. One drug from each group is prescribed.

There are variations in combinations, depending on the needs of the patient and the preferences of the supervising transplant unit.

Antimetabolites prevent the immune system from making T and B cells. Mycophenolate mofetil (MMF or Cellcept) is being used increasingly in place of azathioprine (Imuran). MMF side effects include nausea, diarrhoea and low white blood cell count. Azothioprine side effects are low white blood cell count, bone marrow suppression, liver abnormalities and nausea.

Calcineurin inhibitors inhibit expansion of cells that regulate rejection. Cyclosporine (Neoral) and tacrolimus (Prograf or FK506) are the main drugs in this group. Side effects of cyclosporine include nephrotoxicity, headache, tremor, hyperkalaemia, photosensitivity, gingival hyperplasia and hirsutism. Tacrolimus is at least as effective as cyclosporine in preventing acute rejection and has proved to be effective as a rescue therapy for refractory acute rejection. Side effects are similar to that of cyclosporine, with the exception of gingival hyperplasia and hirsutism.

Steroids specifically prevent expansion of cells that regulate rejection. Prednisolone side effects include obesity, diabetes, osteoporosis, increased cholesterol levels, loss of lean muscle, cataracts and mood swings.

Newer immunosuppressive agents are evolving, with efforts to reduce the nephrotoxicity of calcineurin inhibitors and metabolic toxicity of steroids. Improved longevity of HT recipients means prolonged immunosuppression and consequent use of drugs to prevent or treat long-term complications of immunosuppressive agents, such as infection, obesity, hypertension, hyperlipidaemia, renal insufficiency, diabetes, osteoporosis, gout and malignancies. All immunosuppressive drugs contribute to the risk of malignancy. Risk factors for malignancy are multifactorial and include impaired immunoregulation, a synergistic effect with other carcinogens, such as nicotine or ultraviolet light exposure, and oncogenic viruses such as the Epstein–Barr virus and the papilloma virus. There is a high incidence of lymphoproliferative diseases, skin and lip cancers, and Kaposi's sarcoma in transplant patients, compared with the general population (Lindenfield *et al.*, 2004).

Does reinnervation occur?

Functionally significant reinnervation has not been demonstrated so far (Givertz *et al.*, 1997). Reinnervation is frequently demonstrated, but mainly for sympathetic efferents. The extent of reinnervation increases with time but is variable. It is more likely to occur in young patients, where there was faster uncomplicated surgery and where there is a low frequency of rejection (Bengel *et al.*, 2002). The standard technique leaves around 50% of parasympathetic nerve branches intact in the original atria, so that there are fewer stimuli to reinnervate the donor atria (Bernardi *et al.*, 1998). Therefore, spontaneous reinnervation is an uncommon outcome for patients after transplant. If there is any reinnervation it is most likely to occur many years after surgery.

Contraindications to exercise for heart transplant recipients

Exercise professionals should be aware of situations where exercise is contraindicated for HT recipients until the problem is treated or is stabilised. Contraindications include the following:
• Active infection
• Moderate-to-severe rejection
• Metabolic abnormality
• Any other unstable cardiac problem
• Hypertension, resting systolic blood pressure >200 mm Hg or diastolic blood pressure >110 mm Hg; on exercise systolic pressure >250 mm Hg or diastolic blood pressure >120 mm Hg

Signs of rejection

Rejection is detected by endomyocardial biopsy. The patient will have three biopsies whilst still an inpatient, but the procedure can be carried out on an outpatient basis, following discharge. The biopsy procedure takes about half an hour. Under radiological control, a catheter is introduced into the right internal jugular vein, local anaesthetic having been first administered at the biopsy site. The catheter is advanced down the superior vena cava to the right side of the heart through the tricuspid valve and into the right ventricle. Five to six samples of tissue are obtained and subsequently examined for signs of cellular infiltration.

There is a greater tendency for rejection to occur during the early period after transplant, until the patient's antirejection therapy has been optimised, rather than later in the postoperative course. Consequently, biopsies are carried out weekly for the first 3 weeks postoperatively and then gradually less frequently, as rejection is found to be contained by immunosuppressive drug therapy, which must continue lifelong. Eventually, the patient may only have a biopsy once every 6 months. Patients are informed, usually within 24 hours of the result of the biopsy, so that drug therapy can be optimised at the earliest opportunity, should rejection occur. Any patient involved in a rehabilitation programme can then advise the supervising therapist and have exercise curtailed accordingly.

Grading of rejection in heart transplant recipients
Rejection is graded according to an internationally agreed system as follows:
• Grade 0 denotes no rejection present.
• Grades 1A and 1B are regarded as mild rejection, where there is cellular infiltration of the myocardium but no signs of myocyte damage.

• Grades 2 and 3A are moderate rejection, where there are signs of myocyte damage.
• Grades 3B and 4 denote severe rejection, myocyte damage and necrosis. Clinicians may note signs of right ventricular dysfunction with elevated jugular venous pressure. More severe rejection may be associated with signs of left heart failure and left ventricular dysfunction (Pope *et al.*, 1980).

Signs and symptoms of rejection may be apparent to the patients who will have been educated to recognise and self-monitor themselves for them. Signs include the following:
• A rise in temperature above 37°C, which is sustained
• Ankle swelling, general fluid retention and decreased urine output
• Sudden weight gain of 2 kg or more over 2 consecutive days
• Shortness of breath on exertion
• Generally feeling unwell
• Mood swings
• Fatigue at a level of exercise that does not normally cause a problem
Patients with acute cellular rejection may notice symptoms of fatigue or shortness of breath. Daily weight and temperature are documented by the patients who should report any signs that worry them to the transplant centre.

Similarly to the low adherence with home spirometry measurements, non-adherence to self-monitoring for signs and symptoms was found to be low. De Geest *et al.* (2005) found that non-adherence was ranged between 22 and 59%. Exercise professionals should encourage the patients to be diligent in their self-monitoring and to seek advice and medical attention in time.

Modification of exercise in rejection
Exercise rehabilitation should be discontinued during severe acute rejection. At this time the myocardium is oedematous and subject to cellular infiltration and myofibre injury. Exercise is restricted in order to limit permanent damage to the myocardium. During an episode of moderate rejection, exercise should be maintained at current levels without progression and it should be progressed slowly during periods of mild rejection (Badenhop, 1995; Kavanagh, 1996; Keteyian, 1989).

Exercise and health behaviour change for heart transplant recipients

As for any CR participant, adherence to healthy behaviours over time is needed for the benefits to be accrued. For HT recipients to achieve optimal benefit from the transplant, the patient and family require considerable support and encouragement to maintain their ongoing healthy regimens. It could be argued that the HT recipients have greater needs than other

cardiovascular groups. The HT patients require lifetime attention to the following:
• Lifetime drug therapy concordance with particular emphasis on immunosuppressive medications
• Constant monitoring of signs and symptoms of rejection
• Adherence to healthy diet

(De Geest *et al.*, 2005).

In addition, HT recipients are often found to be more physically inactive after transplant than other CR groups. Some of the reasons for inactivity after surgery include the following:
• Real or perceived barriers including side effects of immunosuppressive therapy
• Doubts about the expected benefits
• Fear that physical activity may precipitate rejection
• A sense of negative well-being

(Evangelista *et al.*, 2005).

(See Thow, 2006, Ch. 8, in addition to long-term cognitive exercise behaviour interventions including exercise consultation.) Exercise professionals must be aware of the added burdens on this group of lifetime health and medication regimes and provide ongoing lifetime support to patients and families.

Key messages

• Heart transplantation is becoming more successful with 5-year survival in excess of 65%.
• Due to pre-surgical heart failure many HT patients are deconditioned prior to CR.
• Due to denervation transplant patients have altered heart rate responses to exercise.
• Exercise can have many positive effects and counteract the side effects of the immunosuppressive medications that these patients must take for their lifetime.
• HT patients will need access to phase IV to maintain lifetime exercise.
• HT patients must be diligent in self-monitoring.
• HT patients need continued psychological monitoring and health behaviour support.

Summary and conclusions

Exercise rehabilitation is an integral part of the management of HT recipients and is a safe and effective way to increase exercise tolerance, decrease potential complications and maximise the outcome of the operation for the patient and the cost-effectiveness of a transplant programme. HT recipients require support to maintain many lifetime therapeutic regimens, including self-monitoring and immunosuppressive medications. These added demands can put considerable pressure on patient and family. Support and health behaviour interventions need to be sustained for this group of cardiac patients.

References

Ainsworth, B.E., Haskell, W.L., Whitt, M.C., *et al.* (2002) Compendium of physical activities: an update of physical activity codes and MET intensities. *Medicine and Science in Sports and Exercise*, 32(Suppl), S498–516.

American College of Sports Medicine (ACSM) (2003) *Exercise Management for Persons with Chronic Diseases and Disabilities*, 2nd edn. Leeds: Human Kinetics.

American College of Sports Medicine (ACSM) (2006) *Guidelines for Exercise Testing and Prescription*, 7th edn. Baltimore, MD: Lippincott, Williams & Wilkins.

Aziz, T., Burgess, M., Khafagy, R., *et al.* (1999) Bicaval and standard techniques in orthotopic heart transplantation: medium-term experience in cardiac performance and survival. *Journal of Thoracic and Cardiovascular Surgery*, 118(1), 115–22.

Badenhop, D.T. (1995) The therapeutic role of exercise in patients with orthotopic heart transplant. *Medicine and Science in Sport and Exercise*, 27(7), 975–84.

Banner, N., Guz, A., Heaton, R., *et al.* (1988) Ventilatory and circulatory responses at the onset of exercise in man following heart or heart-lung transplantation. *Journal of Physiology*, 399, 437–49.

Banner, N.R., Patel, N., Cox, A.P., *et al.* (1989) Altered sympathoadrenal response to dynamic exercise in cardiac transplant recipients. *Cardiovascular Research*, 23(11), 965–72.

Bengel, F.M., Ueberfuhr, P., Hesse, T, *et al.* (2002) Clinical determinants of ventricular sympathetic reinnervation after orthotopic heart transplant. *Circulation*, 106, 806–31.

Bernardi, L., Valenti, C., Wdowczyck-Szulc, J. (1998) Influence of type of surgery on the occurrence of parasympathetic reinnervation after cardiac transplantation. *Circulation*, 97, 1368–74.

Bjarnason-Wehrens, B., Mayer-Berger, W., Meister, E.R., *et al.* (2004) Recommendations for resistance exercise in cardiac rehabilitation. Recommendations of the German Federation for Cardiovascular Prevention and Rehabilitation. *European Journal Cardiovascular Prevention and Rehabilitation*, 11(4), 352–61.

Borg, G.A.V. (1998) *Borg's Perceived Exertion and Pain Scales*. Champaign, IL: Human Kinetics.

Braith, R.W., Limacher, M.C., Mills, R.M., *et al.* (1993a) Exercise-induced hypoxemia in heart transplant recipients. *American College of Cardiology*, 22, 768–76.

Braith, R.W., Limacher, M.C., Leggett, S.H., *et al.* (1993b) Skeletal muscle strength in heart transplant recipients. *Journal of Heart and Lung Transplant*, 12(6 Pt 1), 1018–23.

Braith, R.W., Mills, R.M., Jr, Wilcox, CS., *et al.* (1996) Fluid homeostasis after heart transplantation: the role of cardiac dennervation. *Journal of Heart Lung Transplant*, 15(9), 872–80.

Braith, R.W., Welsch, M.A., Mills, R.M., *et al.* (1998) Resistance exercise prevents glucocorticoid-induced myopathy in heart transplant recipients. *Medicine in Science Sports and Exercise*, 30, 483–9.

Braith, R.W., Wood, C.E., Limacher, M.C., *et al.* (1992) Abnormal neuroendocrine responses during exercise in heart transplant recipients. *Circulation*, 86, 1453–63.

Brubaker, P.H., Brozena, S.C., Morley, D.L., *et al.* (1997) Exercise-induced ventilatory abnormalities in orthotopic heart transplant patients. *Journal of Heart and Lung Transplant*, 16(10), 1011–17.

De Geest, S., Dobbels, F., Fluri, C., *et al.* (2005) Adherence to the therapeutic regimen in heart, lung and heart-lung transplant recipients. *Journal of Cardiovascular Nursing*, 20(5S), S88–98.

Eisen, H.J. (2003) Hypertension in heart transplant recipients: more than just cyclosporine. *Journal of American College of Cardiology*, 41, 433–4.

el-Gamel, A., Yonan, N.A., Grant, S., *et al.* (1995) Orthotopic cardiac transplantation: a comparison of standard and bicaval Wythenshawe techniques. *Journal of Thoracic Surgery*, 109(4), 721–30.

Givertz, M.M., Hartley, L.H., Colucci, W.S. (1997) Long term sequential changes in exercise capacity and chronotropic responsiveness after cardiac transplantation. *Circulation*, 96, 232–7.

Grant, S.C., Khan, M.A., Faragher, E.B. (1995) Atrial arrhythmias and pacing after orthotopic heart transplantation: bicaval versus standard atrial anastomosis. *British Heart Journal*, 74(2), 149–53.

Haskell, W.L., Savin, W.M., Schroeder, J.S., *et al.* (1981) Cardiovascular responses to handgrip isometric exercise in patients following cardiac transplantation. *Circulation Research*, 48(6 Pt 2), 1156–61.

Haykowsky, M., Eves, N., Figgures, L., *et al.* (2003) Early initiation of aerobic and resistance training improves peak aerobic power, leg-press maximal strength and distance walked in six minutes in recent cardiac transplant recipients. *Journal of Heart and Lung Transplant*, 22, S179.

Hertz, M.I., Taylor, D.O., Trulock, E.P., *et al.* (2002) The registry of the international society of heart and lung transplantation: nineteenth official report-2002. *Journal of Heart and Lung Transplant*, 21, 950–70.

Kao, A.C., Van Trigt, P., Shaeffer-McCall, G.S., *et al.* (1995) Allograft diastolic dysfunction and chronotropic incompetence limit cardiac output response to exercise two to six years after heart transplantation. *Journal of Heart Lung Transplant*, 14, 11–22.

Karapolat, H., Eyigör, S., Zoghi, M., *et al.* (2007) Comparison of hospital supervised exercise versus home based exercise in patients after orthoptic heart transplant: effects on function capacity, quality of life, and psychological symptoms. *Transplant Proceedings*, 39(5), 1586–90.

Kavanagh, T. (1996) Physical training in heart transplant recipients. *Journal of Cardiovascular Risk*, 3(2), 154–9.

Kavanagh, T., Yacoub, M.H., Mertens, D.J., *et al.* (1986) Marathon running after cardiac transplantation: a case history. *Journal of Cardiopulmonary Rehabilitation*, 6, 16–20.

Kavanagh, T., Yacoub, M.H., Mertens, D.J., *et al.* (1988) Cardiorespiratory responses to exercise training after orthotopic cardiac transplantation. *Circulation*, 77, 162–71.

Keteyian, S., Ehrman, J., Fedel, F., *et al.* (1989) Exercise following cardiac transplantation. *Sports Medicine*, 8(5), 251–9.

Kobashigawa, J.A., Leaf, D.A., Lee, N. (1999) A controlled trial of exercise rehabilitation after heart transplantation. *New England Journal of Medicine*, 340, 272–7.

Lampert, E., Mettauer, B., Hoppeler, H. (1996) Structure of skeletal muscle in heart transplant recipients. *Journal of American College of Cardiology*, 28, 980–84.

Leon, A.S. (2000) Exercise following myocardial infarction: current recommendations. *Sports Medicine*, 29(5), 301–11.

Lindenfield, J., Miller, G.G., Shakar, S.F., *et al.* (2004) Drug therapy in the heart transplant recipient. *Circulation*, 110, 3734–44.

Mancini, D.M., Eisen, H., Kussmaul, W., *et al.* (1991) Value of peak exercise oxygen consumption for optimal timing of cardiac transplantation in ambulatory patients with heart failure. *Circulation*, 83, 778–86.

Mancini, D.M., Walter, G., Reichek, N. (1992) Contribution of skeletal muscle atrophy to exercise tolerance and altered muscle metabolism in heart failure. *Circulation*, 85, 1364–73.

Marconi, C., Marzorati, M. (2003) Exercise after heart transplantation. *European Journal of Applied Physiology*, 90, 250–59.

Mudge, G.H., Goldstein, S., Addonizio, L.J., *et al.* (1993) 24th Bethesda conference: cardiac rehabilitation. Task Force 3: recipient guidelines/prioritization. *Journal of the American College of Cardiology*, 22, 21–31.

Myers, J., Gullestad, L., Vagelos, R., *et al.* (1998) Clinical, hemodynamic and cardiopulmonary exercise test determinants of survival in patients referred for evaluation of heart failure. *Annals of Internal Medicine*, 129(4), 286–93.

Pate, R.R., Pratt, M., Blair, S.N., *et al.* (1995) Physical activity and public health: a recommendation from the Centres for Disease Control and Prevention and the American College of Sports Medicine. *Journal of the American Medical Association*, 273, 402–7.

Pflugfelder, P.W., Purves, P.D., McKenzie, F.N., *et al.* (1987) Cardiac dynamics during supine exercise in cyclosporine treated orthotopic heart transplant recipients: assessment by radionuclide angiography. *Journal of the American College of Cardiology*, 10(2), 336–41.

Physiotools (2005) *Cardiovascular and Flexibility Exercise.* Finland. Available from http://www.toolsrg.com.

Pope, S.E., Stinson, E.B., Daughters, S.T., *et al.* (1980) Exercise responses of the denervated heart in long term cardiac transplant recipients. *American Journal of Cardiology*, 46, 213–18.

Robson, S.C., Furniss, S.S., Heads, A., *et al.* (1989) Isometric exercise in the denervated heart: a Doppler echocardiographic study. *British Heart Journal*, 61, 224–30.

Rochus, P., Von Duvillard, S.P., Jutta, L., *et al.* (2004) Effect of high-volume and intensity endurance training in heart transplant recipients. *Medicine and Science in Sports and Exercise*, 36(12), 2011–16.

Sarsam, M.A.I., Campbell, C.S., Yonan, N.A. (1993) An alternative surgical technique in orthotopic cardiac transplantation. *Journal of Cardiac Surgery*, 8(3), 344–9.

Savin, W.M., Haskell, W.L., Schroeder, J.S., *et al.* (1980) Cardiorespiratory responses of cardiac transplant patients to graded, symptom-limited exercise. *Circulation*, 62, 55–60.

Scherer, S. (1999) Rating of perceived exertion: development and clinical applications for physical therapy exercise testing and prescription. *Cardiopulmonary Physical Therapy*, 10, 143–58.

Schmidt, A., Pleiner, J., Bayerle-Eder, M., *et al.* (2002) Regular physical exercise improves endothelial function in heart transplant recipients. *Clinical Transplantation*, 16(2), 137–43.

Schwaiblmair, M., von Scheidt, W., Uberfuhr, P., *et al.* (1999) Lung function and cardiopulmonary exercise performance after heart transplantation. *Chest*, 116, 332–9.

Scottish Intercollegiate Guidelines Network (SIGN) (2002) *Cardiac Rehabilitation – A National Clinical Guideline, No. 57*. Edinburgh: SIGN.

Shephard, R.J., Kavanagh, T., Mertens, D.J., *et al.* (1996) The place of perceived exertion ratings in exercise prescription for cardiac transplant patients before and after training. *British Journal of Sports Medicine*, 30(2), 116–21.

Stewart, K.J., Badenhop, D., Brubaker, P.H. (2003) Cardiac rehabilitation following percutaneous revascularization, heart transplant, heart valve surgery, and for chronic heart failure. *Chest*, 123, 2104–11.

Stratton, J.R., Kemp, G.J., Daly, R.C. (1994) Effects of cardiac transplantation on bioenergetic abnormalities of skeletal muscle in congestive heart failure. *Circulation*, 89(4), 1625–31.

Taylor, D.O., Edwards, L.B., Boucek, M.M. (2005) Registry of the international society for heart and lung transplantation: twenty-second official adult heart transplant report – 2005. *Journal of Heart and Lung Transplant*, 24, 945–55.

Tegtbur, U., Busse, M.W., Jung, K., *et al.* (2005) Time course of physical reconditioning during exercise rehabilitation late after heart transplantation. *Journal of Heart and Lung Transplantation*, 24(3), 270–74.

Thow, M.K., McGregor, C., Rafferty, D. (2004) A study of the fitness levels of phase IV men. *European Journal of Cardiovascular Prevention and Rehabilitation*, 11(1), 61.

Thow, M.K., Rafferty, D., Kelly, H. (2008) Exercise motives of long term phase IV cardiac rehabilitation participants. *Physiotherapy*, 94(4), 281–5.

UKTSSA (2007) *United Kingdom Transplant Support Service Authority*. Bristol, UK. Available from www.uktransplant.org.uk (accessed 10 December 2007).

Ulubay, G., Sevinc Sarnc, U., Atilla, S., *et al.* (2007) Assessing exercise performance after heart transplantation. *Clinical Transplantation*, 21(3), 398–404.

Uretsky, B.F., Kormos, R.L., Zerbe, T.R. (1992) Cardiac events after heart transplantation: incidence and predictive value of coronary angiography. *Journal of Heart and Lung Transplant*, 11(3), S45–51.

Ville, N., Mercier, J., Varray, A. (1998) Exercise tolerance in heart transplant patients with altered pulmonary diffusion capacity. *Medicine and Science in Sports and Exercise*, 30, 374–9.

Whaley, M.H., Thomas, W.M., Kaminsky, L.A. (1997) Reliability of perceived exertion during graded exercise testing in apparently healthy adults. *Journal of Cardiopulmonary Rehabilitation*, 17(1), 37–42.

Yusuf, S., Theodoropoulos, S., Mathias, C.J. (1987) Increased sensitivity of the denervated heart to isoprenaline both before and after beta-adrenergic blockade. *Circulation*, 75(4), 696–704.

6   Comorbidity and Ageing

Mhairi Campbell and Hilary Dingwall

Chapter outline

Comorbidity is a term used when an individual is diagnosed with more than one chronic condition. For cardiac rehabilitation (CR) exercise professionals this is an increasing problem. Twenty-six per cent of people with a long-standing condition have three or more problems (Department of Health, 2004b). This highlights the growing complexity of providing care for these individuals. Comorbidities give the exercise professional in CR an additional challenge to assess and provide the most appropriate and most effective individualised programme. This chapter aims to cover three of the most common comorbidities in more detail and the effects of the ageing process than that in Thow (2006, pp. 36–7, 119–29) and to highlight practical measures for applying the art and science of CR in the presence of other comorbidities and ageing.

Coronary heart disease (CHD) tends to be an age-related condition, with the majority of patients presenting with CHD being 50 years or older. In addition to comorbidities and chronic conditions, this section looks at the ageing process and factors the exercise professional working in CR should take into account when prescribing exercise for the older adult.

This chapter covers the following:
• Peripheral arterial disease
• Arthritis
• Ageing

Pathophysiology and incidence of peripheral arterial disease

Atherosclerosis can present not only as coronary heart disease (CHD) but also as peripheral artery disease (PAD). Together, they contribute to a pathological spectrum of diseases involving both coronary and non-coronary circulation (Chan, 2004) but with the same pathological process of deposition of atheroma in the medial wall of the artery.

Peripheral vascular diseases (PVDs) do not have a specific agreed meaning (Fowkes, 2007). However, for the purpose of this chapter the definition of PAD will be 'atherosclerosis of the distal aorta and/or lower limb arteries causing arterial narrowing or disruption of blood flow in the legs'. The most common symptom of PAD is intermittent claudication (IC), which is characterised as lower limb muscle pain, brought on by exercise and relieved by rest (not unlike the presentation of stable angina). This is stage II of a four-stage classification called the Fontaine classification (SIGN, 2006). The location of the pain relates to the anatomical level of disease, but is most commonly felt in the calf muscle, normally reflecting disease in the femoropopliteal segment (SIGN, 2006).

Recording the prevalence of PAD is problematic, as only a small proportion of patients with this condition seek treatment or attend hospital. The Scottish Health Survey (2003), which included questions based on the Edinburgh Claudication Questionnaire, produced the following statistics:
• Prevalence of intermittent claudication increases with age and is more common in women than in men.
• Overall rates for men and women were 2.8 and 3.5%, respectively.
• In those aged over 75 years this increased to 8.9% for men and 6.9% for women.
• IC is more prevalent in those with a history of cardiovascular disease, and 40% of IC sufferers have angina, and of those presenting to hospital, between 38 and 58% have evidence of CHD.

(Fowkes, 2007).

Interestingly, Belch (2003) made epidemiological projections for the population with IC in Europe and North America and suggested prevalence rates of 16% in those over 55 years of age, which is significantly higher than rates in the Scottish Health Survey (2003). This projected higher level in the US was confirmed by the American Heart Association (AHA, 2007), which recently estimated prevalence at 12–20% in those over 65 years of age. These recognised experts predict that this will be a significant and increasing problem for health care providers.

IC and PAD are likely to be much more common than simply for those who have a formal diagnosis via a primary care general practitioner or a vascular specialist. This has implications for clinicians in assessing, designing and delivering CR programmes to ensure that programmes are individualised to the needs of the patient with PAD. It is likely that exercise leaders in CR will encounter patients who describe symptoms that could be attributed to PAD/IC but who have had no formal diagnosis.

Worryingly, PAD has a number of negative effects on its sufferers. In the population older than 55 years, PAD usually indicates diffuse and significant arterial disease (Belch, 2003). Patients with IC often have a progressive reduction in quality of life, despite literature suggesting that most patients improve or stay about the same in terms of the actual IC severity. SIGN (2006) cites evidence that although measurement of ankle brachial pressure index in claudicants deteriorates three times faster than in non-claudicants, the overall deterioration is still only 0.09 mm Hg over 5 years.

The level for PAD diagnosis is <0.9 mm Hg, meaning that there may only be a deterioration of 10% over 5 years for this marker. The Scottish Physiotherapy Amputee Research Group (SPARG, 2002) states that IC symptoms have only been found to be progressive in 25% of people, with 75% of the patient's symptoms stabilising and remaining constant. Some individuals find their symptoms resolve without any intervention. It could be assumed that the reduction in quality of life that IC sufferers experience may be related to a progressive decline in overall fitness, resulting from reduced activity, for example walking shorter distances and walking more slowly.

The main risk for individuals with PAD tends not to be critical limb ischaemia leading to amputation, which occurs in 1% of individuals, but of the associated risk of fatal or non-fatal cardiovascular event (AHA, 2007; SIGN, 2006). Those with PAD have a four- to fivefold increased risk of suffering a cardiovascular disease (CVD) event. This corresponds to a two to three times higher mortality risk (AHA, 2007), with 63% of deaths being the result of CHD (Regensteiner and Hiatt, 2002). This suggests that concomitant CHD and PVD, whether symptomatic and diagnosed or not, negatively impact on each other.

It would therefore seem sensible for any patient with PAD to undergo full cardiac and risk factor screening prior to entering an exercise programme, which for the purposes of this chapter would be normal practice, since we are discussing these patients in the context of also having CHD and participating in a CR programme.

Focusing on the CR perspective, a West of Scotland study (Thow *et al.*, 2003) looked at levels of non-cardiac conditions within the phase III exercise component of eight programmes. Of the 701 patients included, 40 were recorded as having diagnosed with PVD (5.7%), which would fit with rates from the Scottish Health Survey (2003), previously referenced in the chapter. However, cognisance should also be given to the possibility of underdiagnosis, as only 25% of patients in US are undergoing treatment. Another study (Zoghbi *et al.*, 2004) of 409 CR patients found that 74 had PVD, a level of 15%. They then broke these figures down further by looking at patient risk stratification, using the AACPVR (2004) guidelines. They found that the lowest risk group had an incidence of 6.9%; the intermediate, 10.5%; and the highest, 23.5%. This is likely to concur with what exercise professionals now find in the CR patient population: higher risk, complex patients with multiple comorbidities, which can negatively impact on each other.

Recommended treatment for PAD centres on risk factor reduction and symptom control, similar to that for CHD. Cigarette smoking and diabetes are thought to play a significant role in PAD and are particularly strong risk factors (AHA, 2007). There is, however, lower quantity and lower quality evidence relating risk factor treatments to improved cardiovascular outcomes in PAD, but professional consensus supports extrapolation of evidence from CHD studies (Regensteiner and Hiatt, 2002). SIGN (2006) makes its strongest level recommendations on the use of statin, antihypertension and antiplatelet pharmacological therapies and glycaemic control. Due to the lack of higher level evidence, it makes lower level recommendations on smoking cessation, weight control, weight reduction and exercise. Interestingly, there is no mention of physical activity within section 2 of SIGN guideline 89 (SIGN, 2006) for PAD, although it is strongly recommended as a treatment for IC in section 4. Peak exercise performance is known to be significantly reduced in individuals with claudication, at 50% of age-matched non-claudicants (Regensteiner and Hiatt, 2002). The omission of physical activity in the risk reduction section may be due to a lack of research specifically looking at physical inactivity as a risk factor or a lack of evidence on the impact of physical activity and exercise on cardiovascular outcomes in this population. This is highlighted by Garg *et al.* (2006), who concluded from their study that IC patients with higher physical activity levels had lower mortality and event rates, but called for further research to establish the effect of interventions on survival. However, since there is general agreement around the commonality between PAD and CHD, it could be hypothesised that similar benefits could be gained from an exercise-based rehabilitation programme for those with PAD in the present CR patient group.

Benefits of exercise for IC and PAD

Exercise as a treatment for IC is well documented, and there is strong evidence of its benefits (Brandsma *et al.*, 1998; Leng *et al.*, 2000; SIGN, 2006). The benefits include the following:
- Increased pain-free walking distance
- Increased maximum walking distance
- Improved self-reported walking ability
- Quality of life (SIGN, 2006 promotes caution in interpreting the current quality of life evidence and states that further research is needed)
In addition, it should be noted that the Cochrane Collaboration paper (Leng *et al.*, 2000) evaluating exercise for IC found only 15 trials, 5 of which were excluded from analysis, meaning that the total sample size of their meta-analysis was only 250 patients. Within the methodology of the trials, the exercise regimes differed but all used the common activity of walking.

Proposed mechanisms of the physiological benefit of exercise include the following:
- Increased capillary density
- Increased distribution of blood flow to the legs especially to the microcirculation
- More effective distribution of blood flow to the legs
- Improved rheological characteristics of the blood:
  - Decreased fibrinogen levels
  - Decreased plasma viscosity

• Decreased reliance on anaerobic metabolism through increased muscle metabolism efficiency
• Increased cardiorespiratory fitness
• Biomechanics – increased gait efficiency via increased step length (which can be reduced in claudicants)
• Increased pain tolerance, coupled with an increase in confidence and self-efficacy to increase the amount or intensity of walking/exercise undertaken

(Leng *et al.*, 2000; SPARG, 2002).

Exercise therapy has been suggested in the Cochrane Review by Leng *et al.* (2000) to compare favourably with angioplasty in terms of cost and also to have significantly better outcomes after 6 months. This applies particularly to treatment of atherosclerosis of the superficial femoral artery. Exercise confers less mortality risk, which is approximately 4%, compared to surgery, which carries an almost 20% adverse mortality rate. Although exercise is recommended as a treatment for IC, SPARG (2002) and SIGN (2006) acknowledge that there seems little in the way of standard provision or promotion of this treatment. Services for rehabilitation for PAD and IC have yet to be established in much of the UK. A physiotherapy-led service has been established in Lanarkshire, which includes exercise and CVD management (Physiotherapy Frontline, 2008). The benefits available to these patients will not be achieved without access to appropriate exercise prescription.

Assessment for IC and PAD

For patients with PAD, a number of additional factors can be included in a comprehensive CR assessment:
• Is this diagnosed IC or are symptoms highly suggestive? Could it be something else?
• IC is stage II of the Fontaine classification. The evidence for exercise benefit also relates to stage II. Subjective assessment should include questioning to ascertain that the individual's PVD is not at a stage beyond this. Stage III is characterised by rest or nocturnal pain, and stage IV by necrosis or gangrene. This is not unlike the symptom questioning undertaken to ascertain the stability of a CHD patient's angina. Patients with pain at rest or nocturnal pain should probably not be participating in an exercise programme, but should, if appropriate, be redirected to their vascular consultant or primary care physician. Safety to exercise requires that the symptoms of IC should have been stable for a minimum of 3 months according to studies reviewed by the SPARG (2002).
• There should be discussion of the patient's approach to symptom management. Do they avoid activities that bring on symptoms?
• Are they on any medications (as mentioned earlier in this chapter) for symptom control? Are they concordant with that medication?

• Subjectively assess the patients' tolerance of their IC pain when prescribing their individual programme to enhance compliance.
• What is their main limiting factor? Is the IC more likely to be limiting than their CHD? If so, conduct a functional capacity outcome measure to establish a baseline, related to this limiting factor, in order to demonstrate improvement resulting from their programme of exercise. All trials included in the Cochrane Review (Leng *et al.*, 2000) used treadmill testing, but this will not always be applicable in the clinical setting. Using the usual outcome measure, for example shuttle walking test (SWT) (Singh *et al.*, 1992), could be sufficient, with minimal adaptation to capture specific measures of pain onset distance and maximum walking distance. Figure 6.1 shows a record sheet of a shuttle walk test for IC and PVD assessments.

LEVEL	HR	RPE	Shuttles	POD
1			1. 2. 3.	
2			4. 5. 6. 7.	
3			8. 9. 10. 11. 12.	
4			13. 14. 15. 16. 17. 18.	
5			19. 20. 21. 22. 23. 24. 25.	
6			26. 27. 28. 29. 30. 31. 32. 33.	
7			34. 35. 36. 37. 38. 39. 40. 41. 42.	
8			43. 44. 45. 46. 47. 48. 49. 50. 51. 52.	
9			53. 54. 55. 56. 57. 58. 59. 60. 61. 62. 63.	
10			64. 65. 66. 67. 68. 69. 70. 71. 72. 73. 74. 75.	
11			76. 77. 78. 79. 80. 81. 82. 83. 84. 85. 86. 87. 88.	
12			89. 90. 91. 92. 93. 94. 95. 96. 97. 98. 99. 100. 101.102.	

Limiting factor: Leg pain/angina/sob/fatigue/Other (please circle)

Pain onset distance (POD):_____metres

Maximum walking distance:_____metres

Recovery heart rate: 1 minute _____ 2 minutes _____

Figure 6.1 Sample record of shuttle walking test including IC baseline and outcome data. (Adapted from Singh *et al.* 1992.)

• Assessment of IC limitation could also be implemented on a treadmill using a non-incremental steady speed protocol, a 6-minute walking test or endurance shuttle walk test. These may be more sensitive to show improvements in performance related to IC symptoms, since the measures are distance related (pain onset distance and maximum walking distance) and the speed increases of the incremental shuttle walk test are removed.

• Goal setting could include specific walking distance targets built around levels determined from the functional test.

Exercise prescription for IC and PAD

The main features of the exercise prescription for this group of patients can be found in the companion text to this book: *Exercise Leadership in Cardiac Rehabilitation* (Thow, 2006, p. 127). They are summarised in Table 6.1. This follows the FITT (frequency, intensity, time and type) exercise prescription principles (ACPICR, 2006).

It is important that the exercise professional aims to optimally meet the needs of this specific group of patients within their existing CR programmes.

Evidence suggests that supervised exercise is more effective than unsupervised for these patients (Bendermacher *et al.*, 2006). Therefore, encouragement should be given to the individual to attend a structured, supervised class. The potential reasons for this successful approach are as follows:

• The supervised groups mostly use treadmill walking, which can be delivered at a constant, externally paced, specified workload, likely to be higher than normal walking on level ground at an internally paced speed.

• This higher workload is likely to lead to greater cardiovascular improvement.

• Supervision could confer greater adherence to the exercise prescription, and the exercise participation measured and monitored.

Table 6.1 Summary of exercise prescription from exercise leadership in cardiac rehabilitation.

Frequency	Three to five times per week
Intensity	Nudging level of onset of pain 3–4 on RPE
Type	Walking
	Stepping
	Cycling
	Rowing
	Circuit aerobics
	Swimming
Time	Short periods increasing as tolerated

• The group dynamic and exercise leadership could enhance compliance by offering encouragement and motivation, which may not be available during unsupervised exercise.

(Bendermacher *et al.*, 2006).

Exercise intensity

As with any cardiovascular rehabilitation exercise programme the intensity of the individual exercise prescription has to be correct to confer benefit, and in the case of the PAD patient this intensity depends on whether the programme aims to achieve cardiovascular fitness improvement, IC symptom improvement or both. To gain IC improvement the intensity will depend on the individual, but evidence suggests they should be working to near-maximal pain (Bendermacher *et al.*, 2006; Gardner and Poehlman, 1995; SPARG, 2002). Gardner and Poehlman (1995) suggest in their meta-analysis that the claudication pain end point accounted for 55% of the improvement in distance to onset of pain, 40% improvement in maximum pain level. Thus, 'nudging' into pain was the most important component for producing improvement in pain-free walking distance. Although exercise CR professionals do not normally take patients into pain thresholds for the benefit of this group, this is where the skills of the exercise CR professionals are important. They need to explain clearly to the patient the reasons for the encouragement of this practice, and probably to offer more encouragement and support during the exercise session for this group of patients.

The use of a pain scale as a method of self-monitoring in addition to, or instead of, an exertion-focused rate of perceived exertion (RPE) (Borg, 1998) scale could be helpful. An example is shown in Table 6.2.

The patient should try and work at level 3 or 4 on the scale. The aim is for pain to subside between exercises or at least during an active recovery component that takes the focus away from the lower limbs. If the pain rises above 5, then allow the patient to recover sufficiently for it to drop back to 3 or below.

There is a balance to be struck in practical rehabilitation delivery. The evidence supports the best benefit to patients when training at the higher pain level, but since this may compromise compliance, the exercise professional must take a pragmatic approach. A more acceptable level of intensity (i.e. less painful) may have a less pronounced benefit specifically for PAD. However, if the patient is more likely to drop out and be excluded from the other benefits, including other physical, psychological and social gains from exercise-based rehabilitation, then the needs of that patient have not been met. The American College of Sports Medicine (ACSM, 2006) suggests 3–5 minutes of leg activity, with recovery. This exercise recovery pattern is built up from 35 minutes to continuous activity of 50 minutes. The exercise professional should gauge each patient's pain tolerance and

Table 6.2 Borg RPE CR-10 scale.

0	Nothing at all	'No pain'
0.3		
0.5	Extremely weak	Just noticeable
1	Very weak	
1.5		
2	Weak	Light
2.5		
3	Moderate	
4		
5	Strong	Heavy
6		
7	Very strong	
8		
9		
10	Extremely strong	'Max pain'
11		
•	Absolute maximum	Highest possible

Borg (1998).

reaction to exercise, incorporating joint decision, behaviour change and goal-setting strategies into the programme.

Type of exercise
Similarly, the mode of exercise should be addressed. Much of the evidence is based on treadmill walking, which may not even be an option for rehabilitation programmes if treadmills are not available. Other weight-bearing lower limb exercise has been shown to be effective, as has lower and upper limb cycle ergometry.

An interval circuit with periods at higher levels of leg work to a level of leg pain, which also includes upper limb and resistance training, should provide an exercise session that is likely to be well tolerated by the patient, be effective and also fit with the common circuit-based class structure within traditional CR. If the aim within an individual's CR programme is to improve overall exercise capacity, as it will be with most patients, the mode of exercise by which the patient can achieve the appropriate target heart, for the time period required, should be utilised. This is likely to be those that cause less IC pain than promoted for optimum improvement in IC symptoms and likely to comprise non-weight-bearing exercise.

The usual warm-up and cool-down components of the CR class may pose a challenge to the IC patient due to its repetitive, constant, mostly lower limb nature. Modifications will need to be made, and a non-weight-bearing or partial weight-bearing warm-up may be more appropriate for this group.

Frequency and duration elements

The recommended frequency and duration elements of exercise for this group that are recommended are greater than are typically offered by most CR programmes in the UK. The best results are gained by supervised exercise three times a week for a minimum of 6 months.

Total walking duration (including rests) should start at a minimum of 30 minutes, with the aim of increasing to 60 minutes as a maximum (SPARG, 2002).

From a practical and resource point of view, this 6-month period is unlikely to be realistic for most CR exercise professionals to provide, without development of integrated models or partnerships with primary care, leisure and council services, secondary care and health board/authority to provide long-term phase IV programmes. There is no specific reference in any of the literature reviewed to the setting of any rehabilitation programme for PAD, but it could be assumed that the same principles of providing a menu of options dependent on patient's needs be applied, as would be the case for the patient with CHD alone.

Key points for exercise provision for IC and PVD are as follows:
• Establish a baseline and set appropriate goals based on IC as the main presenting condition, if it is the limiting factor.
• Consider the individuals' tolerance to their IC pain when designing their programme.
• Consider a non-weight-bearing or partially non-weight-bearing warm-up exercise.
• Include walking as a significant component, but also include upper and lower limb ergometry, resistance training and interval training format.
• Offer extra support and motivation to patients who are being encouraged to exercise to a level of IC pain.
• Supervised exercise should be encouraged as the most effective option.

Arthritis and incidence

There are over 100 arthritic conditions. The most common are osteoarthritis (OA) and rheumatoid arthritis (RA) which are discussed in this chapter.

Arthritis and related conditions affect millions of people worldwide and place an ever-growing burden on society. More than 7 million adults in the UK (15% of the population) have arthritis-related health problems (ARC, 2002). In the US the estimated arthritis prevalence is 20% of the population or 46 million adults, and it is the leading cause of disability in the US (US Department of Health and Human Services, 2007b). Arthritis is more common in women, and in the 65–74 age group, it is reported to be twice as prevalent in women (Office for National Statistics, 2007).

In the UK, total costs of health and social care, lost-working days and benefits paid total £5.5 billion (ARC, 2002). In the US 29.3% (20.5 million)

45- to 64-year-olds report doctor-diagnosed arthritis, rising to 50.0% of persons aged above 65 (US Department of Health and Human Services, 2007).

OA is a degenerative condition affecting the joint cartilage, which thins and tears. It also affects the underlying subchondral bone, resulting in incongruous joint surfaces. The body's attempts to repair the damaged bone often result in osteophyte formation. The knee is the most commonly affected weight-bearing joint, and the small joints of the hand the most common overall. Key features include the following:

- Pain on motion
- Stiffness following rest/inactivity
- Muscle weakness
- Muscle or joint capsule contracture
- Mechanical block

(ACSM, 2006; Resnick, 2001).

RA is an inflammatory condition and more specifically an autoimmune disorder, where the joint synovium becomes inflamed and swollen. With this recurrent process the synovium becomes progressively thickened, and joint surfaces and bone degenerate. Knuckles and wrists are the most commonly affected areas. Key features include the following:

- Morning stiffness in affected joints
- Joint deformity and reduced joint mobility
- Loss of function, particularly fine motor skills
- Pain
- Fatigue

In relation to the CR population, arthritis is probably one of the most common comorbidities the exercise professional is likely to see. Thow *et al.* (2003) recorded rates of 16% of the non-cardiac conditions additionally encountered in the programmes surveyed, the most common being chronic or acute musculoskeletal problems (56.8%). More profoundly, in 2005 the US recorded concomitant arthritis in 57.8% of the population with heart disease (US Department of Health and Human Services, 2007a).

As the previous section linked peripheral arterial disease with increased cardiovascular mortality, the evidence for rheumatic diseases also suggests an increased cardiovascular risk by Turesson and Matteson (2007). These authors suggest a link between chronic inflammation, sedentary lifestyles and the morbidity and mortality in patients with rheumatic disorders, particularly in systemic lupus erythematosus and rheumatoid arthritis.

Individuals with arthritis are reported to have reduced levels of physical activity, which could be seen as an expected consequence of living with the disease, with its symptoms and impairments.

Almost 44% of adults with doctor-diagnosed arthritis report no leisure time physical activity, compared with 36% of adults without arthritis (US Department of Health and Human Services, 2007). This concurs with other papers that cite differences between arthritis sufferers and those without arthritis. McEntegart *et al.* (2001), in a Glasgow population, found differences in exercise level, with only 26% of those with RA undertaking regular (once a week, which is well below that needed for health gain) exercise and 34% in those without arthritis. Der Ananian *et al.* (2006) cite similar low exercise levels in arthritis sufferers with 34% being 'completely sedentary' to 26% in those without arthritis. However, as an even greater proportion of people become completely sedentary, these differences may eventually be eliminated. This has already been found in a study that included a wide age range, 20–65 years old, of RA and non-RA individuals where there were no differences in physical activity levels (Turesson and Matteson, 2007). In this study 47% of the RA patients in this study did not meet national physical activity recommendations, again re-enforcing the issue of physical inactivity in both the general and arthritis populations.

There is an emerging 'vicious circle', where physical inactivity increases risk of developing arthritis and doubles the risk of developing CHD, while developing arthritis increases physical inactivity and further increases cardiovascular risk (see Figure 6.2).

Benefits of exercise for arthritis sufferers

The benefits of exercise for arthritis sufferers are generally similar to those recognised for CHD (Westby, 2001):
• Increased muscular strength
• Increased flexibility

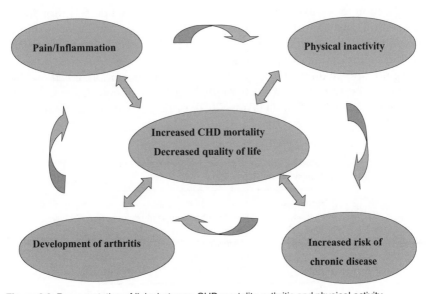

Figure 6.2 Representation of links between CHD mortality, arthritis and physical activity.

- Increased cardiovascular function
- Decreased anxiety and depression
- Improved social activity
- Decreased levels of fatigue
- Decreased or maintained levels of pain
- Possibly decreased or maintained levels of disease activity (Pederson and Saltin, 2006)
- Decreased levels of hospitalisation

Among older adults with knee OA, engaging in moderate physical activity at least three times per week can reduce the risk of arthritis-related disability by 47% (US Department of Health and Human Services, 2007a).

There is little or no evidence for physical activity having a detrimental effect or increasing disease activity (Pederson and Saltin, 2006; Westby, 2001). Finckh *et al.* (2003), however, raise questions in relation to exercise in RA, referring to findings suggesting progressive joint damage caused by higher intensity and high-impact sporting activities, especially in individuals with significant joint damage. Pederson and Saltin (2006) also highlight the lack of evidence around the more seriously affected patients with RA. However, a high-intensity, high-impact programme is most unlikely to be part of the CR 'common sense' approach to exercise, as advocated by the authors and national guidelines (ACPICR, 2006).

How are the benefits achieved: exercise prescription for arthritis

This section focuses on the practical application of that prescription in the CR setting, and identifies considerations the exercise professional should take into account in order to meet the needs of this specific group of patients within their existing programmes.

Again, the main features of the exercise prescription for these patients can be found in the companion text to this book, *Exercise Leadership in Cardiac Rehabilitation* (Thow 2006, p. 127). They are summarised in Table 6.3.

Table 6.3 Summary of exercise prescription from exercise leadership in CR.

Frequency	Three to five times per week
Intensity	60–75% of heart rate maximum
Type	Low impact
	Flexibility
	Strengthening
Time	Overload period of 20–30 minutes

Thow (2006, p. 127).

For a patient with arthritis, there are a number of factors to include in our usual comprehensive assessment, with additional considerations for exercise prescription:

- Which joints are mainly affected?
- What is the range of motion of affected joints? Is it compromised?
- Ascertain if patient has any joint replacements.
- Determine the usual pattern of symptoms, for example morning versus afternoon.
- Establish disease length and severity, particularly to estimate the level and potential of long-term joint damage.
- Usual method and efficacy of pain relief. If current treatment is not enough for the patients to function well during day-to-day activities, they may require a medical review to optimise pain relief in order to permit them to begin an exercise programme.
- Possibility of osteoporosis. Prolonged steroid treatment in the past may have contributed to osteoporosis, along with the chronic inflammatory process and the likely decrease in weight-bearing activity (Pederson and Saltin, 2006).
- Muscle weakness in patients with RA. This can be 30–70% of normal individuals (Pederson and Saltin, 2006).
- Further to this muscle weakness the presence of arthritis can decrease proprioception, flexibility, increase body sway and impair balance (Resnick, 2001). The consequence can be an increased risk of falls. Does the patient have a history of falls or loss of balance?
- The combination of stiffness, weakness, poor mobility and decreased efficiency of movement can result in physical activities having a higher metabolic cost for these patients; that is, they require a higher level of energy expenditure. This could be as much as 50% higher (ACSM, 1998).

Evidence suggests that for both main types of arthritis, exercise prescription is similar for CR patients, but with some differences and adjustments.

The type of exercise suggested for individuals with arthritis encompasses a broad range, including aerobic conditioning, isotonic and isometric strength training, flexibility, balance and coordination (ACSM, 2006; Pederson and Saltin, 2006; Resnick, 2001). The following section discusses each of these types of exercise in relation to CR exercise programmes.

Aerobic conditioning

Aerobic conditioning can safely and effectively be delivered by most of the common modalities recommended in CR, such as walking, swimming, cycling, low-impact circuit aerobics and water-based aerobics.

In land-based exercise, specific consideration should be given to kinetic variables, such as ground reaction forces and joint compression forces by considering the floor or ground surface, for example concrete versus sprung or cushioned flooring, use of cushioning footwear and prescription of low-impact activities. Additionally, shearing and rotary forces should be minimised by encouraging good movement patterns and good exercise technique, coupled with activities that move joints in a single plane, such as walking, which is a primarily saggital plane activity in the lower limbs (Westby, 2001).

However, not all patients, especially those who have had longer duration or more severe arthritis, will be able to tolerate walking or full weight-bearing exercise. Non- or partial-weight-bearing exercise such as cycling is likely to be most appropriate and best tolerated, although weight-bearing exercise has a role to play in maintaining or protecting against loss of bone density (Pederson and Saltin, 2006).

Water-based aerobic activities, where exercise can be carried out in water, are appropriate for arthritis sufferers and can often reduce pain symptoms by decreasing joint compression forces, increasing sensory input from the external water turbulence, pressure and temperature, and muscle relaxation provided by the water buoyancy (Westby, 2001). Further individual advice should be given with regards to swimming, in relation to patients, some of which are considerations we would also give to the CHD patient population (see Thow, 2006, pp. 74–5, 117–18). Levels of skill and technique are important, as swimming will result in a higher intensity exercise for beginners or for those lacking skill in the water. Additionally, risk stratification of CHD patients in relation to water-based exercise should be undertaken. Not all patients are suitable for exercising in this medium, due to the physiological effect of both water pressure and position when swimming on cardiac preload and afterload and the likelihood of a reduction in perceived exertion in water.

Resistance exercise

Care should be taken when introducing any resistance component to a programme that the joints are protected; that is, the surrounding muscles are strong enough to undertake the given exercise without undue joint strain and in some cases gravity or auto-assisted exercise may be most appropriate. For some individuals it may also be necessary to improve strength in a particular area before aerobic exercise can be undertaken and the aim of increasing cardiovascular fitness can be achieved. Strength training is particularly important in RA to combat the consequences of the skeletal muscle wasting found in RA (Pederson and Saltin, 2006; Resnick, 2001). Isometric strengthening exercise is suggested due to the lack of movement at the joint, thereby reducing risk of exacerbation of pain and inflammation (Resnick, 2001). Care should be taken in prescribing isometric exercises for cardiac patients due to the likelihood of the adverse physiological effects in this population (as discussed in Thow, 2006, Ch. 4, p. 114). However, to fully meet the needs of the patient with arthritis, practitioners may wish to include this type of exercises for specific muscle groups. This suggestion may require enhanced levels of supervision, monitoring and coaching to prevent Valsalva (breath holding), which could theoretically be more easily precipitated here than by isotonic strengthening exercises. Practitioners need to decide the feasibility of this within their programmes.

Flexibility, balance and coordination

Range of motion exercises and stretching routines should ideally be performed daily by people with arthritis and encouraged by the exercise professional if they are not already part of the patient's condition management routine. Flexibility exercise is an integral part of CR exercise, particularly in the cool-down phase when subjects are well warmed-up. Hyperextension should be avoided, and it is important to ensure that the patient has enough muscle strength to control each movement throughout the range or at point of stretch.

Other additional, possibly complementary components that could be included in an arthritis patient's exercise prescription to best meet their individual needs include the following:
• Gait re-education to improve efficiency of movement and therefore energy expenditure, and to reduce the risk of falls
• Fall practice, which can be incorporated into a class if mat work is included to encourage individuals to learn how to get off the floor in the event of a fall
• Specific balance and coordination activities
However, it has been shown that the more established components of a CR session – circuit aerobic and resistance training – can reduce postural sway and balance, thereby achieving improved mobility and reducing the risk of falling (Resnick, 2001) without the inclusion of the above-suggested 'complementary' activities. We can therefore be reassured that without a huge amount of adaptation we will meet many of the needs of many patients with multiple conditions including arthritis.

Pain management

Pain is a likely symptom for most patients with arthritis. Like patients with PVD they may require extra support to manage this during initiation and to encouragement to adhere to an exercise programme. However, the exercise undertaken should not be to a level that increases an individual's pain overall. Some post-exercise discomfort should probably be expected and the patient reassured about this, but it should not last more than a couple of hours after the session (ACSM, 1997). Additionally, for RA patients exercise should not be undertaken until morning stiffness has eased, and afternoon sessions may be more appropriate. Effective, regular analgesia is important and should always be taken, but the patient should be vigilant not to 'mask' exercise pain by taking extra painkillers. Patients should be informed about this and aspect of exercise, and exercise professionals should check on pain control and pain management at each session.

Key points for exercise provision for arthritis sufferers are as follows:
• Identify specific arthritis-related limitations that can be improved by exercise.
• Design individual patient exercise programmes to address these limitations.
• When considering exercise prescription, aim to limit adverse joint stresses.
• Ensure adequate, regular analgesia.

The ageing process

Ageing is a complex process involving many variables (e.g. genetics, lifestyle factors and chronic diseases) that interact with one another, greatly influencing the manner in which we age (Mazzeo *et al.*, 1998).

The Oxford English Dictionary (2005) defines old age as 'the later part of normal life' and 'the state of being old'. The problem with these definitions is that they do not define the attributes of old age or describe the criteria for each 'part' of normal life. Old age cannot be defined exactly because it does not have the same meaning in all societies. In some parts of the world, people are considered old just because of changes in their social circumstances or activities.

Global demographic trends of older people

The rising number and proportion of aged individuals in the population is a global demographic trend (Martin and Sheaff, 2007). In the US the percentage of people 65 years or over increased from 4% (3 million) in 1900 to 13% (34 million) in 1990. Population experts predict that by 2020 about 17% (50 million) of the population will be over 65 (American Association of Retired Persons, 2007). In the UK the number of people over 65 will increase from 11.4 million in 2006 to 12.2 million in 2011, and will rise to 13.9 million by 2026, reaching 15.3 million in 2031 (Age Concern, 2007). It can be assumed from these projected demographics that we will see many older patients enrolling in CR programmes.

People are living longer healthier lives, and many of the public health-related problems that caused mortality are now under control. Lifestyle changes, public health improvements and improved health care have all combined to extend life expectancy. Advancing age is generally accompanied by a progressive decline in physical activity (Evans and Meredith, 1989). For sometime performance decline was thought to be normal and a necessary consequence of ageing. However, in more recent studies physically active older women were found to have performance patterns of flexibility, balance and agility more similar to younger participants than to older inactive adults (Nakamura *et al.*, 2006). Regular physical activity helps prevent conditions prevalent in 'old age', notably osteoporosis, non-insulin-dependent diabetes, hypertension, ischaemic heart disease, stroke and perhaps some cancers, specifically colon cancer (Young and Dinan, 2005).

Pathophysiology of ageing

As discussed previously, ageing is a complex process involving many variables greatly influencing the manner in which we age (ACSM, 1998; Mazzeo *et al.*, 1998).

Ageing affects cardiovascular response to exercise, muscle mass and strength, bone density, postural stability, flexibility, balance and risk of falling.

Cardiovascular response to exercise

Maximal oxygen uptake (VO_2max) is defined as the maximal volume of oxygen the body can take up and use, based on the following three main physical aspects:
1. The size and strength of the heart
2. The amount of blood a person has and the amount of oxygen the blood can carry
3. The amount of oxygen (VO_2) the muscles can extract from the blood
(Buckley et al., 1999).

VO_2max is known to decrease with age (Heath *et al.*, 1981). After the age of 25, in non-training individuals there is approximately a reduction of 1% per year (Lambert and Evans, 2005). It is unclear if maintaining a high level of activity can slow the rate of decline. However, a highly active person will have a higher value of VO_2max than a sedentary one at each equivalent age. This loss in VO_2max can be attributed to several factors.

There is a decline in maximal cardiac output (CO). CO is the volume of blood pumped by each ventricle per minute, that is the product of stroke volume and heart rate. As maximal heart rate decreases six to ten beats per decade, this is responsible for much of the age-associated decrease in maximal CO (Pollock *et al.*, 1997). Some evidence also highlights that older adults have smaller stroke volumes during maximal exercise (Ogawa *et al.*, 1992). The reduction in stroke volume is attributed to a reduction in preload (the work imposed on the heart before contraction begins and equates to the end-diastolic volume), an increase in afterload (the pressure in the arteries that the heart must overcome to eject the blood from the ventricles) and reduced myocardial contractility (BACR, 2002). Elasticity of all major blood vessels declines naturally with ageing (ACSM, 2001). The increase in afterload is caused by an increase in the total peripheral resistance, approximately 1% per year from the age of 40 onwards (Kenney, 1989).

There is also a reduction in maximal arterial–venous oxygen differ-ence (a-VO_2 difference), the difference in oxygen content between arterial and mixed venous blood. This reflects the amount of oxygen removed by the tissues. This reduction in a-VO_2 difference may be the result of microstructural changes, including myofilament disorganisation and changes in mitochondrial structure and distribution, resulting in reduced oxidative capacity (ACSM, 2001).

Another factor that may indirectly contribute to a loss in VO_2max is actual physical limitation resulting from a sedentary lifestyle, loss of coordination and disabling diseases such as arthritis. The consequence of the decline in VO_2max is that every physical task requires a higher percentage of VO_2max in an older person than a younger one.

A study by Kohrt *et al.* (1991) demonstrated that elderly individuals (aged 67–71) exercising 4 days/week, 45 minutes/day for 9 months to 1 year with exercise intensity gradually increasing from 76% of heart rate maximum to 86% of heart rate maximum will improve VO_2max by 24%. However, such high intensities are not realistic for most of the elderly population, due to decreased motivation and increased risk of injury associated with high-intensity exercise (ACSM, 2001).

Systolic and diastolic blood pressures

Hypertension (persistently high blood pressure) is one of the most common disorders in the UK. Although it rarely causes symptoms on its own, the damage it does to the arteries and the organs they supply can lead to considerable suffering, avoidable deaths and burdensome health care costs (Faculty of Public Health, 2005).

According to the World Health Organization (2002), the global disease burden attributable to a systolic blood pressure (SBP) of 115 mm Hg or above is 20% of all deaths in men and 24% of all deaths in women, 62% of strokes and 49% of CHD and 11% of disability-adjusted life years (WHO, 2002). Worldwide, approximately 50% of the burden of CVD in people aged 30 years and over can be attributed to an SBP of 115 mm Hg or above (WHO, 2002).

Arterial blood pressure is the maximum pressure of the blood exerted on the arterial walls as the ventricles contract (systolic pressure), over the minimum pressure, which is exerted when the heart relaxes between contractions (diastolic pressure). *The British Hypertension Society Guidelines* (2003) recommend blood pressure targets of <140/85 (no diabetes) and <140/80 (with diabetes).

Blood pressure is the product of CO and the amount of resistance to blood flow from the total peripheral resistance within the circulation (BACR, 2002). Blood vessels undergo changes with advancing age, including arterial stiffening and thickening. This is due to an increase in collagen and smooth muscle (Herbert, 2006). As arteries stiffen they resist the flow of blood, especially the pulsatile flow in the large arteries nearest the heart. This resistance is a key factor in rising SBPs with age. Increased afterload resulting from increased peripheral resistance appears to be the primary mechanism for ventricular hypertrophy (Fleg *et al.*, 1988). Further away from the heart, resistance to the smoother flow of blood in the arteries governed by the arterioles determines peripheral vascular resistance.

Pulmonary function

Several changes occur in the thorax and lungs that have an adverse effect on function. These changes are mainly the result of loss of elasticity of the lungs and chest wall. As lung tissue loses its elasticity due to loss of collagen, there is an increase in the work involved in breathing. Both vital capacity (VC, the total volume of air expelled after maximal inhalation) and forced expiratory volume (FEV1, the greatest volume of air exhaled in 1 second) decrease, and residual volume (RV, the amount that cannot be exhaled) increases.

Despite these changes, older adults will only have slightly reduced pulmonary function and during exertion will increase ventilation by increasing their rate of breathing rather than the depth. If required, advice on breathing control should be given by the exercise professional where appropriate.

Bone

Women begin to lose bone at age 30, and will lose about 20% by the age of 65 and 30% by the age of 80. Men begin to lose at the age of 40 onwards, and will lose 10–15% by the age of 70 and 20% by the age of 80 (ACSM, 2006). Weight-bearing exercise and muscle contraction are particularly important for older women to maintain bone health.

Strength

Muscle function decreases approximately 25% by the age of 65 (ACSM, 2006). This decline in strength generally begins at the age of 30 and will be more marked in women than in men, and will be greater in the lower limbs than the upper limbs (BACR, 2002). Therefore, it is appropriate to include resistance exercise training in a comprehensive exercise programme.

Joints and flexibility

Both flexibility and range of movement decline with age. Combined with reductions in strength, this may result in an increased likelihood of falls and exacerbate arthritic problems. Incorporating flexibility exercises into the programme reduces this risk. As flexibility is a key feature of the CR cool-down, this aspect is well addressed in CR programmes.

Body composition

Age brings a reduction in lean body mass and an increase in body fat (American Council on Exercise, 1998). Both men and women gain weight, and this is generally a result of an imbalance of calorie intake and energy expenditure. Changes in metabolism also contribute to weight gain.

The increased energy expenditure associated with exercise and improved muscle-to-fat ratio assists weight management (ACSM, 2006).

Balance

Balance, reaction times and motor coordination deteriorate with age. When combined with deterioration in hearing and eyesight, these changes have been shown to increase the likelihood of falls by 35–40% in adults over 60 (ACSM, 2001). Participants may have difficulty hearing/seeing instructions, and this can lead to anxiety or loss of confidence. The exercise leader must consider the class environment in order to be sensitive to the specific needs of participants. Although age reduces motor skills, it is important to incorporate motor skills into CR exercise programmes to ensure practice and skill rehearsal. Studies have found that exercise of a mixture of weight-bearing activities and balance can reduce falls by 22% in those aged between 62 and 95 years (Lord *et al.*, 2003). Thus, balance, weight-bearing exercise and motor skills require practice and should be part of all CR programmes to maintain and improve balance, reaction and motor coordination.

Cardiovascular exercise prescription for older adults

Despite age-related changes to the cardiovascular system, the benefits of cardiovascular training are similar in older and younger people (BACR, 2006).

The FITT principle of progressive overload is applicable to the older adult (BACR, 2006). However, consideration must be given to the person's exercise history, medical history, medications, exercise environment (e.g. temperature, lighting and floor surface) and personal likes and dislikes (ACSM, 2001).

Frequency of exercise for older subjects

If exercise is performed at a lower intensity then it is advisable to be performed on most days of the week.

Intensity

When prescribing exercise intensity age, related predicted maximum heart rates should be used only as a rough guide (BACR, 2006). The standard typical target heart rate zone was originally established with healthy, younger, more active individuals, and has possibly been wrongly applied across larger cross sections of the population (Buckley *et al.*, 1999). Actual heart rate maximums may vary from the estimate by as much as ±20 beats/min (BACR, 2006). Therefore, the use of RPE (Borg, 1998), along with heart rate, should be encouraged. However, it is recommended that training intensities should initially be at the lower end of the normal prescription and progression should be more gradual (BACR, 2006). If using heart rate to set an intensity level for older adults, a range between 60 and 75% maximum heart rate is recommended (ACSM, 2006).

Research has shown that even a minimal amount of regular physical activity has a significant effect on aspects of health (Department of Health, 2004). It may therefore be more appropriate to prescribe lower intensity exercise, as this will allow an elderly person to cope and may improve compliance.

Time

Older adults should be encouraged both to accumulate at least 30 minutes of functional accumulated activity, such as housework, gardening and stair climbing, on most days of the week and to build up to sustained periods of exercise of up to 20–30 minutes of continuous activity.

Accumulating shorter 5- or 10-minute bouts at different times of the day, for example, will enable those who find it difficult to maintain longer durations of exercise to achieve health benefits. Once the older person can sustain 10 minutes they can try to increase the duration. Exercise duration should be increased before intensity in order to avoid injury and encourage compliance.

When designing an exercise session for older adults, it is important to consider that peripheral blood flow, such as to the legs, decreases with ageing (Wilmore and Costill, 1994). A study by Wahren *et al.* (1974) shows a reduction of between 10 and 15% in blood flow to the exercising muscles in middle-aged athletes at any given work rate, compared with well-trained young athletes. Redistribution of blood to the skeletal muscles therefore takes longer, as does the length of time required to increase the coronary supply in order to meet the physiological demands of exercise. With this in mind, older adults should be encouraged to extend the length of their warm-up (BACR, 2006).

Type

The AHA (1992) states that activities such as walking, hiking, cycling, rowing and swimming, as well as sports such as tennis, football and basketball, are all beneficial when performed regularly and that the most apparent effects will be gained at exercise intensities exceeding 50% of the person's exercise capacity. The most favourable type of exercise will be client dependent. Older adults will often have at least one comorbidity, and exercise programmes must be designed to accommodate these conditions. As already discussed, hypertension is very common in older adults, and therefore when designing an exercise programme for this client group, it is essential that the effects of exercise on blood pressure are taken into consideration.

When a person undertakes a bout of exercise, SBP will rise in direct proportion to increased exercise intensity (Wilmore and Costill, 1994). The use of the upper body, as opposed to the lower body, will result in a greater rise in SBP. This greater rise in SBP is due to the smaller muscle mass and smaller vascular system of the upper body, compared with the lower. The difference in size means that there is increased resistance to blood flow, that is increased peripheral resistance and therefore greater resistance for the heart to overcome (Wilmore and Costill, 1994), if a person exercises using their upper body.

This increased resistance has implications for the exercising heart muscle and the amount of oxygen it will consume. The rate pressure product or double product is an indirect measure of myocardial oxygen consumption, and is the product of heart rate and SBP divided by 100. With arm exercises, as the SBP increases so will the rate pressure product, resulting in a greater workload for the myocardium.

Resistance training for older adults

There is a gradual loss of muscle mass and strength between middle and late age in men and women. This causes a reduction in muscle strength in older person and inactive individuals. Sedentary older individuals can show both a loss in muscle mass and an increase in subcutaneous fat. Not only do older adults lose muscle mass but both slow (type 1) and fast (type 2) fibres become smaller and may even be lost completely. This may be because they lose their nerve supply. An elderly person's muscles will contract more slowly and this loss of speed can contribute to the loss of power, which begins in middle age (Harridge and Young, 1997).

Loss of strength is greater in women than in men and generally greater in the lower compared to the upper body. Older adults are able to carry out activities that require only moderate amounts of muscle strength, for example postural support, but are deficient when higher force is required. Loss of strength can lead to a reduction in quality of life, as simple tasks become more difficult, for example walking, stair climbing, dressing activities and standing up from a chair or toilet. As muscles contract more slowly they may have insufficient power to correct any loss of balance, and therefore older adults are more likely to fall. As muscle can act as a protective cushion over, for example the hipbone loss of muscle mass around this area can increase the likelihood of a fracture.

Exercise considerations for muscle strength

In the past, exercise guidelines did not recommend resistance training for rehabilitation programmes for older adults. However, in 1990s the ACSM recognised that strength training was an essential part of a well-designed training programme. A scientific advisory was published in 2000 by the AHA, recommending resistance training and highlighting its benefits to health in individuals with or without CVD (Blair and Morrin, 2000). Now it is widely recognised that strength training is effective in improving strength, balance, functional capacity and bone density in older adults

(Fiatarone *et al.*, 1990). Resistance training will enable elderly individuals to perform activities of daily living with greater ease and allow them to take part in occupational and recreational activities, thus allowing older adults to retain their independence.

Frequency
The ACSM recommends that resistance training be performed at least twice a week, with at least 48 hours rest between sessions. However, a report by Verrill (2001) suggests that training three times per week on non-consecutive days is ideal for older adults, but also low level exercises, for example hand weights or elastic bands, may be performed once daily.

Intensity
When considering intensity, several variables should be considered, for example number of sets, number of repetitions and amount of resistance. The ACSM (2000) guidelines recommend that one set of eight to ten exercises are performed using all major muscle groups – quadriceps, hamstrings, gluteals, pectorals, latissimus dorsi, deltoids and abdominals, with each set involving 10–15 repetitions.

Different techniques can be used to determine resistance training load. The one repetition maximum (1 RM) or maximal voluntary contraction can be used, but care should be taken when using this technique, as it can be associated with increases in blood pressure. Eventually the level should be set at 40–60% of the individual's 1 RM. Another way to determine the correct resistive load may be by using an acclimation technique, where the workload starts with a lighter weight and is gradually increased every 1 or 2 weeks.

Anyone undertaking a resistance training programme should be encouraged to use the correct breathing technique, breathing out with the effort. The Valsalva manoeuvre (forced exhalation against a closed glottis) should be avoided, as it can produce a marked increase in blood pressure. The increase in peripheral resistance and reduction of blood flow through the muscles, as well as an increase in intrathoracic pressure, may reduce venous return and stroke volume. These changes will increase myocardial oxygen demand when CO is reduced (ACSM, 2001). The Borg (1998) scale is often considered a more useful tool during resistance exercise. The patient should not experience greater exertion during resistance exercise than in the aerobic component. On the 6–20 Borg (1998) point scale, participants should be advised to work between 11 'fairly light' and 14 'somewhat hard' (ACSM, 2001).

Time
It is recommended that older adults complete their total body resistance programme in 20–30 minutes. Significant strength gains can be seen in individuals with fewer sets and lighter loads (ACSM, 2001).

Sessions lasting any longer may lead to increased dropout rates, smaller additional gains in strength, increased fatigue and a potential increased risk of musculoskeletal injuries (Gordon *et al.*, 1995).

Type

The modality will depend on numerous factors. Accessibility, convenience and enjoyment should all be taken into consideration to encourage adherence. The use of machines to train, as opposed to free weights, is advisable as resistance machines require less skill, provide joint protection, allow lower resistances to be used and increased by smaller increments, and allow the participant to more easily control the exercise range (ACSM, 2000).

Other activities, such as gardening, housework and walking, may also help to maintain muscular strength.

Flexibility

Flexibility consists of adequate range of movements of a single or multiple joints and depends on bone, muscle and connective tissue structure and function.

As people get older, there is a general loss in flexibility as a result of several factors, including disuse, deterioration of the joint structures and degeneration of collagen fibres. Flexibility is important in maintaining an adequate level of musculoskeletal function, balance and agility in older adults. Adequate flexibility should also improve functional capacity and reduce the likelihood of injuries and falls (ACSM, 2000).

Exercise considerations for flexibility

Frequency

The guidelines state that a stretching exercise programme should be carried out at least two to three times per week (ACSM, 2000), and it is recommended that short stretches are incorporated into a warm-up for older adults in order to reduce the likelihood of injury by preparing the muscle for movements that will be performed during the conditioning component of the class. During the cool-down, developmental stretches should be included, that is stretches held for 15–30 seconds targeting the major muscle groups, for example hip, back, knee, upper trunk and neck. For subjects who have had coronary artery bypass grafting, stretches for the pectoral muscle should be considered to prevent adaptive shortening post-surgery.

Intensity, time and type

Preparatory stretches should be incorporated into a warm-up and held for between 8 and 10 seconds. Developmental stretches should be held for

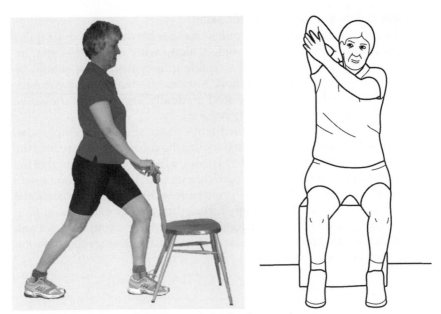

Figure 6.3 Examples of home flexibility exercises (Physiotools, 2005, © Finladn).

between 15 and 30 seconds. The amount of stretch should not cause pain, but should be taken to the point of mild discomfort and held, with four repetitions of each muscle group (ACSM, 2000). The participants should be encouraged to breathe normally, ease into the stretch and not to bounce. The exercise leaders and assistants should be observing participants' performance for position and quality of the exercise and should correct poor technique.

Yoga is recommended and is helpful in improving flexibility, with some yoga practitioners dedicating 30–45 minutes every day to stretching (ACSM, 2001). In addition, home programmes can be designed to incorporate flexibility exercise. A good method is using material from Physiotools (Physiotools, 2005). The exercise professional can design a suitable standing or sitting routine that the patient can carry out at home (see Figure 6.3).

Motor skills

As a result of loss of neurones and a loss of connective tissue networks in the brain over time, numerous changes occur to the central and peripheral nervous systems, for example loss of neural function, slower conduction velocities and reaction times, which drop by 15% by the age of 70 (ACSM, 2001). This slowing down of processing and responding to a stimulus means that balance, reaction times and motor skills will be affected. This slow-down, combined with a loss of strength, makes falls more likely in older people.

Exercise considerations for motor skills

To reduce the likelihood of falls, quick changes between moves or quick changes in direction should be avoided, along with any exercise that involves crossing over the legs, for example grapevines. These should be excluded or used with great caution. Movements that require dynamic standing balance should be introduced gradually, and support should be provided if required and gradually reduced.

T'ai Chi, a sequence of slow meditative exercises, which emphasises the gentle rotation and stretching of the spine, has been shown to reduce the risk of multiple falls (Wolf *et al.*, 1996). It can also be introduced as part of the CR programme and will provide participants with benefits of motor skill and balance. When designing CR programmes, the exercise professional should provide classes that not only focus on cardiovascular conditioning where exercise machines are predominantly used, for example cycles and treadmills, but also aim to intersperse activities that challenge coordination and motor skills (see Figure 6.4).

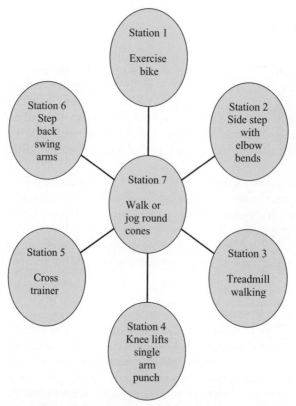

Figure 6.4 Circuit format with mix of cardiovascular equipment (stations 1, 3 and 5) interspersed with stations that incorporate cardiovascular and motor skill (stations 2, 4 and 6).

Special senses

Both hearing and vision will be affected by age. Numerous changes occur in all parts of the ear with ageing. Hearing is at its most efficient at the age of 10, and then gradually deteriorates. Sensitivity to high frequencies, which contribute to the understanding of speech, declines with age. There is a decline in the speed and accuracy of the auditory orienting reflex (which helps locate sound) (Herbert, 2006). Vestibular abnormalities caused by hardening of the bones of the inner ear can result in dizziness. Changes to the structure and function of the eyes can cause deterioration to vision. If older adults suffer from swollen feet and ankles, it may result in reduced proprioception sensitivity. This could lead to problems with foot placement and again increase the likelihood of a fall.

As a result of these changes to the special senses, older clients can feel anxious about attending any form of exercise programme, and all these factors must be taken into consideration when designing any exercise programme for older adults.

Exercise considerations for special senses

Music is often used in an exercise setting. However, when working with older adults it is important that the volume does not obscure the instructor's voice.

The instructor should be as visible as possible to all participants in the class; a combination of visual and verbal cues should be used and all instructions should be clear and precise (see Chapter 7 for more on teaching in Thow, 2006).

Medication considerations

With age there is a greater likelihood of developing a chronic disease. Many of the diseases suffered by older adults will be treated with medication to improve quality of life and help to encourage independence. As older adults are more likely to suffer from numerous health problems, the amount of medication taken by the individual may also increase. The Department of Health (2001) established that older people receive more prescriptions per head than any other group. *Polypharmacy* is defined as the practice of prescribing four or more medications for the same individual. Ziere *et al.* (2006) found that fall risk is associated with polypharmacy. For exercise instructors, a detailed knowledge of all medications is not required. However, it is the responsibility of the instructor to have a basic understanding of the common drugs, and their side effects, they may encounter when working with older adults. If issues arise on medication, consultation with the pharmacy or a pharmacist is essential.

Outcome measures

One of the most commonly used outcome measures of aerobic functional capacity in the cardiac population is the SWT. This test was first described by Singh *et al.* (1992) and was originally designed for patients with chronic obstructive pulmonary disorders. The test is simple to use, requires very little equipment and can be undertaken by the majority of cardiac patients. It starts at a very slow speed and is suitable for older adults. The test can be used to determine appropriate exercise intensities and assist in designing an individualised home walking programme as well as measuring changes in functional capacity before and after training.

The 6-minute walk test (Butland *et al.*, 1982) may be a more sensitive outcome measure for elderly patients. It is safe, easy to administer, better tolerated and reflects activities of daily living better than other walking tests, for example the SWT (Enright *et al.*, 2003).

The elderly mobility scale (Smith, 1994) may also be used to assess improvements in function. It measures locomotion, balance (functional reach) and key position changes (sit to stand, lie to sit, sit to lie, stand with and without support).

The Tenetti test (Tenetti, 1986) is another easily administered test that measures gait and balance.

Exercise behaviour change for older adults

It is well documented that older people participate in less activity, and as people age they become more sedentary, more so for women than for men (see Figures 6.5 and 6.6). Thus, assisting and motivating exercise

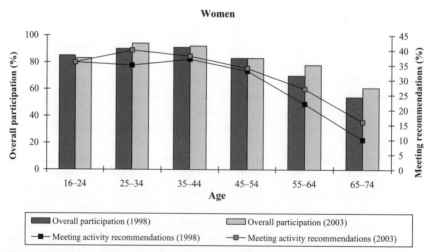

Figure 6.5 Female participation levels reaching recommended levels of 30 minutes of moderate exercise most days of the week (Scottish Executive, 2002).

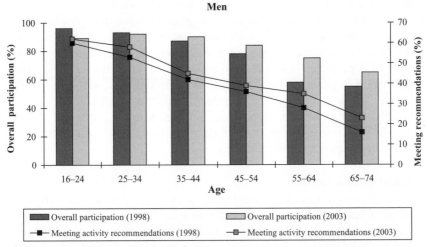

Figure 6.6 Male participation levels reaching recommended levels of 30 minutes of moderate exercise most days of the week (Scottish Executive, 2002).

participation in older people may be more challenging than in younger subjects.

In addition to the cognitive behaviour change that is normally used in CR (see Thow *et al.*, 2003, Ch. 8), many other factors should be considered when helping older adults start and adhere to habitual exercise. Laventure and Skelton (2007) suggest that these factors are viewed as three categories:

1. Personal characteristics
2. Programme factors
3. Environmental factors

Personal characteristics

These include the older person's perceptions and beliefs, which are often affected by ageist stereotyping, negative images and myth. His or her current health status and concern about pain and discomfort can be a barrier. Finally, the person's previous exercise experience can influence his or her perceptions of exercise. Confidence and self-efficacy are strong indicators of uptake and adherence to exercise for older people. Exercise professionals in CR must build on the older person's confidence and ability to take part in the exercise programme. Sensitive application of cognitive behaviour change should be employed, exploring expectations and goals, overcoming real and perceived barriers and providing regular positive feedback (Laventure and Skelton, 2007; Thow, 2006).

Programme factors

For older adults the types of exercise and variety are important. As CR is delivered in a 'menu-based' approach (SIGN, 2002), a variety of class formats and exercises should be given. Older adults favour the more moderate types of exercise. As this is the level of exercise that is delivered in CR, older adults should be easily incorporated into exercise. Furthermore, adherence is more favourable when delivered at low-to-moderate intensities (ACSM, 2006). The skills, enthusiasm and empathy of the exercise leader are recognised as key factors in participation (ACSM, 2006; Laventure and Skelton, 2007). Social support, enjoyment and fun are cited as key adherence and motivation factors for the older CR participant (Thow et al., 2008). CR exercise professionals should facilitate social interaction and create a fun atmosphere in their classes.

Environmental factors

The amount and quality of support is a significant factor in adherence and involvement in exercise in older adults. Many people can provide support to older people, including family, peers and care providers. CR programmes routinely involve the family in health behaviour (SIGN, 2006). Where older people are involved, extra effort to provide support should be employed. The physical environment is important, with time of class, access and parking all cited as barriers to older adult participation (Laventure and Skelton, 2007). Where possible, CR teams should design programmes to address these issues in order to minimise barriers to participation, thus maximising the potential for older people to access exercise and gain the health benefits.

Key messages

• Due to the worldwide demographics there will be many more elderly CR participants.
• Many older CR participants will have comorbidities.

Peripheral arterial disease
• IC as a CVD disorder is present in many CR participants and is on the increase.
• IC is often diagnosed for the first time by CR exercise professionals.
• IC sufferers can progressively reduce levels of activity.
• Cardiovascular risk factor reduction and increasing exercise should be a key feature of rehabilitation for this group.
• Habitual exercise has many favourable effects for PAD sufferers.
• Assessment of IC limitations should be part of a CR assessment.
• Supervised exercise appears to confer grater adherence and improvements in this group.
• Leg pain is the main determinant of exercise intensity.

Arthritis
• Arthritis is very prevalent in the older population.
• Arthritis is one of the most common comorbidities seen in CR.

• Many arthritis sufferers are inactive, contributing to CHD risk.
• Regular exercise improves musculoskeletal and cardiovascular function in this group.
• Musculoskeletal assessment and monitoring should be integrated into the management of CR subjects with arthritis.
• Ground reaction forces and pain management are key variables for this group.

Ageing
• Ageing changes pose many challenges to CR professionals due to altered response to exercise.
• Including exercise prescription for aerobic and strength, balance, motor skills and flexibility are important for older adults.
• Older people are often on many medications.
• Older people have changes in special senses, particularly hearing and vision that can affect exercise.
• Older people are less active and will need sustained support and targeted exercise behaviour change strategies.

Summary and conclusions

There is no doubt that many older adults will be referred to CR. The exercise professionals need to have a knowledge and understanding of the many comorbidities that the older adults will present with and be able to adapt and adjust their classes and exercise prescription. Furthermore, the older adult may not have any apparent copathology, but the consequences of ageing also need to be taken into consideration when delivering safe and effective exercise. Finally, participation and adherence to exercise pose many challenges for the CR exercise professional. Strategies that address the personal programme and environmental factors for this group should be explored for the individual older person.

References

Age Concern (2007) *Statistics on Ageing*. Available from http://www.ageconcern. org.uk (accessed 21 January 2007).

American Association of Cardiovascular and Pulmonary Rehabilitation (AACPVR) (2004) *Guidelines for Cardiac Rehabilitation Program*, 4th edn. Champaign, IL: Human Kinetics.

American Association of Retired Persons (2007) *Statistics of American Adults*. Available from http://www.aarp.org (accessed 18 January 2007).

American College of Sports Medicine (ACSM) (1997) *ACSM's Exercise Management for Persons with Chronic Diseases and Disabilities*. Leeds, UK: Human Kinetics.

American College of Sports Medicine (ACSM) (1998) Position stand: exercise and physical activity for older adults. *Medicine and Science in Sports and Exercise*, 30(6), 992–1008.

American College of Sports Medicine (ACSM) (2000) *Guidelines for Exercise Testing and Prescription*, 6th edn. Baltimore, MD: Lippincott Williams & Wilkins.

American College of Sports Medicine (ACSM) (2001) *Resource Manual for Guidelines for Exercise Testing and Prescription*, 4th edn. Balitmore, MD: Lippincott Williams & Wilkins.

American College of Sports Medicine (ACSM) (2006) *Resource Manual for Guidelines for Exercise Testing and Prescription*, 7th edn. Balitmore, MD: Lippincott Williams & Wilkins.

American Council on Exercise (1998) *Exercise for Older Adults*. Champaign, IL: Leeds: Human Kinetics.

American Heart Association (AHA) (1992) Statement on exercise. Benefits and recommendations for physical activity programs for all Americans. A statement for health professionals by the Committee on Exercise and Cardiac Rehabilitation of the Council on Clinical Cardiology, American Heart Association. *Circulation*, 86, 340–44.

American Heart Association (AHA) (2007) *Peripheral Arterial Disease Statistics*. Available from http://www.americanheart.org (accessed January 2007).

Arthritis Research Campaign (ARC) (2002) *Factfile: Arthritis at a Glance*. Available from http://www.arc.org.uk/about_arth/astats.htm (accessed February 2007).

Association of Chartered Physiotherapists in Cardiac Rehabilitation (ACPICR) (2006) *Standards for the Exercise Component of Phase III Cardiac Rehabilitation*. London: Chartered Society of Physiotherapy.

Belch, J. (2003) Critical issues in peripheral arterial disease detection and management. A call to action. *Archives of Internal Medicine*, 163, 884–92.

Bendermacher, B.L.W., Willigendael, E.M., Teijink J.A.W., *et al.* (2006) Supervised exercise therapy versus non-supervised exercise therapy for intermittent claudication. *Cochrane Database of Systematic Reviews*, Issue 2. Art No.: CD005263. DOI: 10.1002/14651858.CD005263.pub2.

Blair, T., Morrin, L. (2000) *Resistance Training Guidelines. American Heart Association (AHA), American College of Sports (ACSM) and Canadian Association of Cardiac Rehabilitation (CACR) Guidelines for Resistance Training*. Canadian Association of Cardiac Rehabilitation Newsletter.

Borg, G.A.V. (1998) *Borg's Perceived Exertion and Pain Scales*. Champaign, IL: Human Kinetics.

Brandsma, J.W., Robeer, G.B., Van Den Heuvel, S., *et al.* (1998) The effect of exercises on walking distance of patients with intermittent claudication: a study of randomised clinical trials. *Physical Therapy*, 78, 278–88.

British Association for Cardiac Rehabilitation (BACR) (2002) *BACR Exercise Instructors Training Module*, 3rd edn. Leeds: Human Kinetics.

British Association for Cardiac Rehabilitation (BACR) (2006) *BACR Exercise Instructors Training Module*, 4th edn. Leeds: Human Kinetics.

British Hypertension Society Guidelines (2003) *Target Blood Pressure Levels*. UK: Oxbridge Solutions Limited.

Buckley, J., Holmes, J., Mapp, G. (1999) *Exercise on Prescription, Cardiovascular Activity for Health*. Oxford: Butterworth Heinemann.

Butland, R.J.A., Pang, J., Gross, E.R., *et al.* (1982) Two-, six-, and 12-minute walking tests in respiratory disease. *BMJ*, 284, 1607–8.

Chan, A.W. (2004) Expanding roles of the cardiovascular specialists in panvascular disease prevention and treatment. *Canadian Journal of Cardiology*, 20(5), 535–44.

Department of Health (2001) *National Service Framework for Older People*. London: Department of Health.

Department of Health (2004a) *At Least Five a Week: Evidence on the Impact of Physical Activity and Its Relationship to Health*. London: Department of Health.

Department of Health (2004b) *Chronic Disease Management: A Compendium of Information*. London: Department of Health.

Der Ananian, C.A., Wilcox, S., Abbott, J., *et al.* (2006) The exercise experience in adults with arthritis: a qualitative approach. *American Journal of Health Behaviour*, 30(6), 731–44.

Enright, P.L., McBurnie, M.A., Bittner, V., *et al.* (2003) The six minute walk test: a quick measure of functional status in elderly adults. *Chest*, 123(2), 387–98.

Evans, W.J., Meredith, C.N. (ed.) (1989) *Exercise and Nutrition in the Elderly, Nutrition, Aging and the Elderly*. New York: Plenum Press.

Faculty of Public Health (2005) *Easing the Pressure: Tackling Hypertension Is a Toolkit for Developing a Local Strategy to Tackle High Blood Pressure*. London: Faculty of Public Health.

Fiatarone, M.A., Marks, E.C., Ryan, N.D. (1990) High intensity strength training in nonagenarians. Effect on skeletal muscle. *Journal of the American Medical Association*, 263(22), 3029–34.

Finckh, A., Iversen, M., Liang, M.H. (2003) The exercise prescription in rheumatoid arthritis: primum non nocere [comment]. *Arthritis and Rheumatism*, 48(9), 2393–5.

Fleg, J.L, Gerstenblith, G., Lakatta, E.G. (1988) Pathophysiology of the aging heart and circulation. In: *ACSM Resource Manual for Guidelines for Exercise Testing and Prescription*, 4th edn. Balitmore, MD: Lippincott Williams & Wilikins.

Fowkes, F.G.R. (2007) *Peripheral Vascular Disease*. Health Care Needs Assessment Series 3. Available from http://www.hcna.radcliffe-oxford.com/pvd.htm (accessed 20 February 2007).

Gardner, A., Poehlman, E. (1995) Exercise rehabilitation programmes for treatment of claudication pain: a meta analysis. *Journal of the American Medical Association*, 274, 975–80.

Garg, P.K., Tian, L., Criqui, M.H., *et al.* (2006) Physical activity during daily life and mortality in patients with peripheral arterial disease. *Circulation*, 114(3), 242–8.

Gordon, N.F., Kohl, H.W., Pollock, M.L. (1995) Cardiovascular safety of maximal strength testing in healthy adults. *American Journal of Cardiology*, 76(11), 851–3.

Harridge, S.D.R., Young, A. (1997) Skeletal muscle. *Principles and Practice of Geriatric Medicine*, 3rd edn. London: John Wiley & Sons Ltd.

Heath, G., Hagberg, J., Ehsani, A., *et al.* (1981) A physiological comparison of young and older endurance athletes. *Journal of Applied Physiology*, 51, 634–40.

Herbert, R.A. (2006) The Biology of human ageing. In: Redfern, S.J., Ross, F.M. (eds), *Nursing Older People*, 4th edn. Edinburgh, UK: Churchill Livingstone.

Kenney, H.A. (1989) *Physiology of Aging: A Synopsis*, 2nd edn. Chicago: Year Book.

Kohrt, W.M., Malley, M.T., Coggan, A.R., *et al.* (1991) Effects of gender, age and fitness level on response of VO_2 max to training in 60–71 year olds. *Journal of Applied Physiology*, 71, 2004–11.

Lambert, C.P., Evans, W.J. (2005) Adaptations to aerobic and resistance exercise in the elderly. *Reviews in Endocrine and Metabolic Disorders*, 6, 137–40.

Laventure, R., Skelton, D.A. (2007) Breaking down the barriers: strategies to motivate the older client to begin and sustain exercise participation. *Fitness Professionals Magazine*, 42–3.

Leng, G.C., Fowler, B., Ernst, E. (2000) Exercise for intermittent claudication. *Cochrane Database of Systematic Reviews*, Issue 2, Art No.: CD000990, DOI: 10.1002/ 14651858. CD000990.

Lord, S.R., Castell, S., Corcoran, J., *et al.* (2003) The effects of group exercise on physical performance and falls in frail older people in a retirement village a randomised controlled trial. *Journal of the American Geriatric Society*, 51, 1658–92.

Martin, J.E., Sheaff, M.T. (2007) The pathology of ageing: concepts and mechanisms. *Journal of Pathology*, 211(2), 111–3.

Mazzeo, R.S., Cavanagh, P., Evans, W.J., *et al.* (1998) Exercise and physical activity for older adults. *Medicine and Science in Sports and Exercise*, 30, 992–1008.

McEntegart, A., Capell, H.A., Creran, D., *et al.* (2001) Cardiovascular risk factors, including thrombotic variables, in a population with rheumatoid arthritis. *Rheumatology*, 40(6), 640–44.

Nakamura, Y., Tanaka, K., Yabushita, N., *et al.* (2006) Effects of exercise frequency on functional fitness in older adult women. *Archives of Gerontology and Geriatrics*, 44(2), 163–73.

Office for National Statistics (2007) Heart disease and stroke statistics. *Circulation*, 115, 69–171.

Ogawa, T., Spina, W., Martin, W., *et al.* (1992) Effects of aging, sex and physical training on cardiovascular responses to exercise. *Circulation*, 86, 494–503.

Pederson, B.K., Saltin, B. (2006) Evidence for prescribing exercise in chronic disease. *Scandinavian Journal of Medicine and Science in Sports*, 16, 3–63.

Physiotherapy Frontline (2008) The Chartered Society of Physiotherapy Magazine. *Vascular Clinics Roll Out*, 14(10), 9.

Physiotools (2005) *Cardiovascular and Flexibility Exercise*. Finland. Available from http://www.toolsrg.com

Pollock, M., Mengelkoch, L., Graves, J., *et al.* (1997) Twenty year follow up of aerobic power and body composition of older track athletes. *Journal of Applied Physiology*, 82, 1508–16.

Regensteiner, J., Hiatt, W. (2002). Current medical therapies for patients with peripheral arterial disease: a critical review. *American Journal of Medicine*, 112, 49–57.

Resnick, B. (2001) Managing arthritis with exercise. *Geriatric Nursing*, 22(3), 143–50.

Scottish Executive (2002) *Lets Make Scotland More Active: A Strategy for Physical Activity Task Force*. Edinburgh, UK: Crystal Mark.

Scottish Health Survey (2003) *Volume 1: Cardiovascular Disease*. Available from http://www.scotland.gov.uk/resource/doc/76169/0019727.pdf (accessed 3 June 2008).

Scottish Intercollegiate Guidelines Network (SIGN) (2002) *Cardiac Rehabilitation – A National Clinical Guideline No. 57*. Edinburgh, UK: SIGN.

Scottish Intercollegiate Guidelines Network (SIGN) (2006) *Diagnosis and Management of Peripheral Arterial Disease – A National Clinical Guideline No. 89*. Edinburgh, UK: SIGN.

Scottish Physiotherapy Amputee Research Group (SPARG) (2002) *Guidelines for Exercise Therapy for Patients with Intermittent Claudication*. Glasgow, UK: SPARG.

Singh, S.J., Morgan, M.C.D.L., Scott, S., *et al.* (1992) Development of a shuttle walking test in patients with chronic airways obstruction. *Thorax*, 47, 1019–24.

Smith, R. (1994) Validation and reliability of the elderly mobility scale. *Physiotherapy*, 80, 744–7.

Tenetti, M. E. (1986) Performance-orientated assessment of mobility problems in elderly patients. *Journal of the American Geriatrics Society*, 34, 119–26.

The Oxford English Dictionary (2005) 3rd edn, Oxford: Oxford University Press.

Thow, M.K. (ed). (2006) *Exercise Leadership in Cardiac Rehabilitation – An Evidence-Based Approach*. West Sussex, UK: Wiley.

Thow, M.K., Armstrong, G., Rafferty, D. (2003) A survey to investigate the non-cardiac conditions and the physiotherapy interventions by physiotherapists in phase III cardiac rehabilitation exercise programs. *Physiotherapy*, 89(4), 233–7.

Thow, M.K., Rafferty, D., Kelly, H. (2008) Exercise motives of long term phase IV cardiac rehabilitation participants. *Physiotherapy*, 94(4), 281–5.

Turesson, C., Matteson, E.L. (2007) Cardiovascular risk factors, fitness and physical activity in rheumatic diseases. *Current Opinion in Rheumatology*, 19, 190–96.

US Department of Health and Human Services. (2007a) *Arthritis: At a Glance*. National Center for Chronic Disease Prevention and Health Promotion. Available from http://www.cdc.gov/nccdphp/publications/aag/pdf/arthritis.pdf (accessed 12 November 2007).

US Department for Health and Human Services. (2007b) *Statistics of Arthritis*. National Center for Chronic Disease Prevention and Health Promotion. Available from http://www.cdc.gov/arthritis/data_statistics/arthritis_related_statistics.htm (accessed 12 November 2007).

Verrill, D.E. (2001) Strength training for older adults [Special Report]. *Geriatric Times*, 2(4), 26–7.

Wahren, J., Saltin, B., Jorfeldt, L., *et al.* (1974). Influence of age on the local circulatory adaptation to leg exercise. *Scandinavian Journal of Clinical Laboratory Investigations*, Suppl 126, 37–79.

Westby, M.D. (2001) A health professionals guide to exercise prescription for people with arthritis: a review of aerobic fitness activities. *American Journal of Rheumatology*, 6, 501–11.

Wilmore, J.H., Costill, D.L. (1994) *Physiology of Sport and Exercise*, 2nd edn. Champaign, IL: Human Kinetics.

Wolf, S.I., Barnhart, H.X., Kutner, N.G. (1996) Reducing frailty and falls in older persons: an investigation of T'ai Chi and computerised balance training. *Journal of the American Geriatrics Society*, 44, 489–97.

World Health Organization (2002) *Reducing Risks. Promoting Healthy Life. The World Health Report*. Geneva: World Health Organization.

Young, A., Dinan, S. (2005) Activity in later life, ABC of sports and exercise medicine. *British Medical Journal*, 330, 189–91.

Ziere, G., Dieleman, J.P., Hofman, A., *et al.* (2006) Polypharmacy and falls in the middle age and elderly population. *British Journal of Clinical Pharmacology*, 61(2), 218–23.

Zoghbi, G., Sanderson, B., Breland, J., *et al.* (2004) Optimizing risk stratification in cardiac rehabilitation with inclusion of a co-morbidity index. *Journal of Cardiopulmonary Rehabilitation*, 24, 8–13.

Index

6-minute walk test (6 MWT), 84

acute myocardial infarction, 8
age-adjusted maximum heart rate
    (AAMHR), 118
ageing process
  definition, 178
  exercise
    behaviour change in older adults,
      190–92
    cardiovascular, for older adults,
      182–4
    exercise considerations for flexibility,
      186–7
    global demographic trends of older
      people, 178–9
    for motor skills, 187–8
    outcome measures of aerobic functional
      capacity, 190
    resistance training for older adults,
      184–6
    for special senses, 189
  medication, 189
  pathophysiology
    balance, 182
    body composition, 181–2
    bone health, 181
    cardiovascular response to exercise,
      179–80
    joints and flexibility, 181
    strength, 181
    systolic and diastolic blood pressures,
      180–81
Alberti, Sir George, 5
albuminuria excretion, 44
amiodarone, 100, 104

anastomoses, 139
angiotensin-converting enzyme (ACE)
    inhibitors, 81–2
antiarrhythmic versus implantable
    defibrillator (AVID), 105
antimetabolites, 154
antitachycardia pacing (ATP), 108–9
armchair management, 1
arrhythmia. *see also* implantable
    cardioverter defibrillator (ICD)
  and associated ECG profiles, 120
  conditioning component, 127
  defined, 96
  design of exercise programmes, 122–3
  efficiency effect of CR exercise, 123–4
  evidence for cardiac rehabilitation (CR),
    113–14
  during exercise, 97–8
    influencing factors, 98
    performance of patients, 98–100
  types of exercises for, 124–6
arrhythmogenic right ventricular
    cardiomyopathy, 116
arthritis and related conditions
  exercise
    benefits of, 173–4
    regime, 174–8
  incidence, 171–3
Association of Physiotherapists in Cardiac
    Rehabilitation, 15–16
atherosclerosis, 162
autonomic neuropathy, 43
azothioprine, 154

β-blockade therapy, for CHF, 82–3, 100, 119
Bainbridge reflex, 140